# Exercise for Better Bones

Improve Bone Health and Reduce Falls and Fractures
With Osteoporosis-Friendly Exercises for Seniors

**Baz Thompson**

# Table of Contents

**Part 1: The Foundation**      **2**

Introduction . . . . . . . . . . . . . . . . . . . . . . . . . . . . . . . . . . . . . . . . . . . . . . . . . . . . .3

     What is Your Motive? . . . . . . . . . . . . . . . . . . . . . . . . . . . . . . . . . . . . . . . . 3

     My Personal Connection . . . . . . . . . . . . . . . . . . . . . . . . . . . . . . . . . . . . 4

     What is Osteoporosis? . . . . . . . . . . . . . . . . . . . . . . . . . . . . . . . . . . . . . . . 4

     Actions You Can Take. . . . . . . . . . . . . . . . . . . . . . . . . . . . . . . . . . . . . . . 5

     How to Use This Book . . . . . . . . . . . . . . . . . . . . . . . . . . . . . . . . . . . . . . 7

     Hope. . . . . . . . . . . . . . . . . . . . . . . . . . . . . . . . . . . . . . . . . . . . . . . . . . . . . . 9

**Part 2: The Exercises**      **10**

**Chapter 1: Improving Your Balance** . . . . . . . . . . . . . . . . . . . . . . . . . . . **11**

     ***Balance Exercises***

     3 Way Hip Kick . . . . . . . . . . . . . . . . . . . . . . . . . . . . . . . . . . . . . . . . . . . . 13

     Bird Dog . . . . . . . . . . . . . . . . . . . . . . . . . . . . . . . . . . . . . . . . . . . . . . . . . 14

     Foot Taps. . . . . . . . . . . . . . . . . . . . . . . . . . . . . . . . . . . . . . . . . . . . . . . . . 15

     Head Rotation . . . . . . . . . . . . . . . . . . . . . . . . . . . . . . . . . . . . . . . . . . . . 16

     Heel Raises . . . . . . . . . . . . . . . . . . . . . . . . . . . . . . . . . . . . . . . . . . . . . . . 17

     Hip Abductor. . . . . . . . . . . . . . . . . . . . . . . . . . . . . . . . . . . . . . . . . . . . . 18

     Lateral Stepping . . . . . . . . . . . . . . . . . . . . . . . . . . . . . . . . . . . . . . . . . . 19

     Mini-Lunge. . . . . . . . . . . . . . . . . . . . . . . . . . . . . . . . . . . . . . . . . . . . . . . 20

Single Leg Stance . . . . . . . . . . . . . . . . . . . . . . . . . . . . . . . . . . . . . . . . . . . . . . . . . . . . . . . . . . . . . . 21

Sit to Stand . . . . . . . . . . . . . . . . . . . . . . . . . . . . . . . . . . . . . . . . . . . . . . . . . . . . . . . . . . . . . . . . . . . . . 22

Standing Marches . . . . . . . . . . . . . . . . . . . . . . . . . . . . . . . . . . . . . . . . . . . . . . . . . . . . . . . . . . . . . . . 23

Over-the-Shoulder Walks . . . . . . . . . . . . . . . . . . . . . . . . . . . . . . . . . . . . . . . . . . . . . . . . . . . . . . . 24

## Chapter 2: Improving Your Flexibility . . . . . . . . . . . . . . . . . . . . . . . . . . 25

### *Flexibility Exercises*

Breaststroke . . . . . . . . . . . . . . . . . . . . . . . . . . . . . . . . . . . . . . . . . . . . . . . . . . . . . . . . . . . . . . . . . . . . . 27

Calf Stretch . . . . . . . . . . . . . . . . . . . . . . . . . . . . . . . . . . . . . . . . . . . . . . . . . . . . . . . . . . . . . . . . . . . . . . 28

Chest Stretch . . . . . . . . . . . . . . . . . . . . . . . . . . . . . . . . . . . . . . . . . . . . . . . . . . . . . . . . . . . . . . . . . . . . 29

Corner Stretch . . . . . . . . . . . . . . . . . . . . . . . . . . . . . . . . . . . . . . . . . . . . . . . . . . . . . . . . . . . . . . . . . . 30

Inner Thigh Stretch . . . . . . . . . . . . . . . . . . . . . . . . . . . . . . . . . . . . . . . . . . . . . . . . . . . . . . . . . . . . . 31

Kneeling Hip Flexor Stretch . . . . . . . . . . . . . . . . . . . . . . . . . . . . . . . . . . . . . . . . . . . . . . . . . . . . . 32

One Leg Kick . . . . . . . . . . . . . . . . . . . . . . . . . . . . . . . . . . . . . . . . . . . . . . . . . . . . . . . . . . . . . . . . . . . . 33

Prone Heel Squeeze . . . . . . . . . . . . . . . . . . . . . . . . . . . . . . . . . . . . . . . . . . . . . . . . . . . . . . . . . . . . . 34

Side Angle Pose . . . . . . . . . . . . . . . . . . . . . . . . . . . . . . . . . . . . . . . . . . . . . . . . . . . . . . . . . . . . . . . . . 35

Side Kick . . . . . . . . . . . . . . . . . . . . . . . . . . . . . . . . . . . . . . . . . . . . . . . . . . . . . . . . . . . . . . . . . . . . . . . . 36

Superman Pose . . . . . . . . . . . . . . . . . . . . . . . . . . . . . . . . . . . . . . . . . . . . . . . . . . . . . . . . . . . . . . . . . . 37

Supine Hand-to-Big Toe . . . . . . . . . . . . . . . . . . . . . . . . . . . . . . . . . . . . . . . . . . . . . . . . . . . . . . . . 38

## Chapter 3: Improving Your Posture . . . . . . . . . . . . . . . . . . . . . . . . . . . . 39

### *Posture Exercises*

Dead Bug . . . . . . . . . . . . . . . . . . . . . . . . . . . . . . . . . . . . . . . . . . . . . . . . . . . . . . . . . . . . . . . . . . . . . . . 41

Glute Bridge . . . . . . . . . . . . . . . . . . . . . . . . . . . . . . . . . . . . . . . . . . . . . . . . . . . . . . . . . . . . . . . . . . . . 42

Head Press . . . . . . . . . . . . . . . . . . . . . . . . . . . . . . . . . . . . . . . . . . . . . . . . . . . . . . . . . . . . . . . . . . . . . . 43

Isometric Abdominals . . . . . . . . . . . . . . . . . . . . . . . . . . . . . . . . . . . . . . . . . . . . . . . . . . . . . . . . . . . 44

Modified Forearm Side Plank . . . . . . . . . . . . . . . . . . . . . . . . . . . . . . . . . . . . . . . . . . . . . . . . . . . . 45

Shoulder Blade Squeeze . . . . . . . . . . . . . . . . . . . . . . . . . . . . . . . . . . . . . . . . . . . . . . . . . . . . . . . . . 46

Shoulder Rolls . . . . . . . . . . . . . . . . . . . . . . . . . . . . . . . . . . . . . . . . . . . . . . . . . . . . . . . . . . . . . . . . . . 47

Tandem Stand . . . . . . . . . . . . . . . . . . . . . . . . . . . . . . . . . . . . . . . . . . . . . . . . . . . . . . . . . . . . . . . . . . 48

Tandem Walk . . . . . . . . . . . . . . . . . . . . . . . . . . . . . . . . . . . . . . . . . . . . . 49

Tree Pose . . . . . . . . . . . . . . . . . . . . . . . . . . . . . . . . . . . . . . . . . . . . . . . 50

Wall Angels . . . . . . . . . . . . . . . . . . . . . . . . . . . . . . . . . . . . . . . . . . . . . 51

Waxing. . . . . . . . . . . . . . . . . . . . . . . . . . . . . . . . . . . . . . . . . . . . . . . . . . 52

**Chapter 4: Improving Your Strength** . . . . . . . . . . . . . . . . . . . **53**

***Strength Exercises***

Clamshell . . . . . . . . . . . . . . . . . . . . . . . . . . . . . . . . . . . . . . . . . . . . . . 55

Elbow Side Extensions . . . . . . . . . . . . . . . . . . . . . . . . . . . . . . . . . . . 56

Forearm Plank . . . . . . . . . . . . . . . . . . . . . . . . . . . . . . . . . . . . . . . . . . 57

Hammer Curls . . . . . . . . . . . . . . . . . . . . . . . . . . . . . . . . . . . . . . . . . . 58

Hamstring Curls . . . . . . . . . . . . . . . . . . . . . . . . . . . . . . . . . . . . . . . . 59

Lateral Shoulder Raise . . . . . . . . . . . . . . . . . . . . . . . . . . . . . . . . . . . 60

Prone Leg Lifts . . . . . . . . . . . . . . . . . . . . . . . . . . . . . . . . . . . . . . . . . 61

Squats . . . . . . . . . . . . . . . . . . . . . . . . . . . . . . . . . . . . . . . . . . . . . . . . . 62

Standing Push-Up . . . . . . . . . . . . . . . . . . . . . . . . . . . . . . . . . . . . . . 63

Stomping . . . . . . . . . . . . . . . . . . . . . . . . . . . . . . . . . . . . . . . . . . . . . . 64

Upright Rows. . . . . . . . . . . . . . . . . . . . . . . . . . . . . . . . . . . . . . . . . . . 65

Wall Slide . . . . . . . . . . . . . . . . . . . . . . . . . . . . . . . . . . . . . . . . . . . . . . 66

**Chapter 5: Improving Your Cardio**. . . . . . . . . . . . . . . . . . . . . **67**

***Cardio Exercises***

Common Weight-bearing Exercises . . . . . . . . . . . . . . . . . . . . . . . . . . . 69

Less Common Weight-bearing Exercises . . . . . . . . . . . . . . . . . . . . . . . . 70

One More Thing . . . . . . . . . . . . . . . . . . . . . . . . . . . . . . . . . . . . . . . . . 71

**Part 3: The Action Plan**             **72**

**Chapter 6: Exercise Routines**. . . . . . . . . . . . . . . . . . . . . . . . . . . **73**

Week 1: Three Days Training and Two Days CardioYou choose your two rest days. . . . . . . . . . 74

Week 2: Three Days Cardio and Two Days Training ..................................... 75

Week 3: Three Days Training and Two Days Cardio ..................................... 75

Week 4: Three Days Cardio and Two Days Training ..................................... 76

Conclusion ....................................................................... 77

References ........................................................................ 79

# BEFORE YOU START READING

As a special gift, I included a logbook and my book, **"Strength Training After 40"** (regularly priced at $16.97 on Amazon) and the best part is, you get access to all of them for **FREE**.

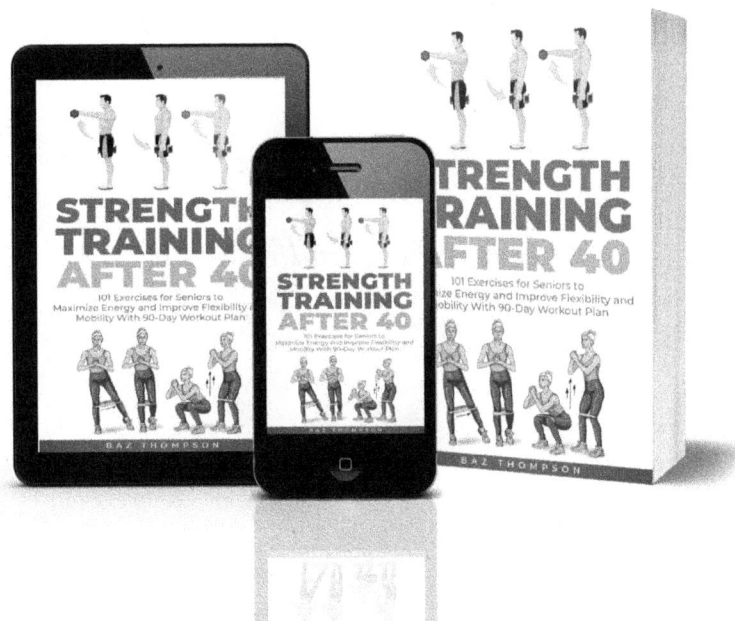

What's in it for me?

◈ 101 highly effective strength training exercises that can help you reach the highest point of your fitness performance

◈ Foundational exercises to improve posture and increase range of motion in your arms, shoulders, chest, and back

◈ Stretches to help you gain flexibility and find deep relaxation

◈ Workout Logbook to help you keep track of your accomplishments and progress. Log your progress to give you the edge you need to accomplish your goals.

SCAN THE QR CODE

# Part 1:
## The Foundation

> *An investment in knowledge
> pays the best interest.*
>
> **Benjamin Franklin**

# Introduction

**W**elcome to your journey toward better bones! This book is all about improving your bone health through exercise and good practices. The goal is to prevent you from breaks, falls, and fractures because of poor balance, flexibility, posture, or strength. You can make a significant impact on your health and well-being through some simple daily choices.

Before we begin incorporating the exercises, let's take a look at why you are reading this book and why I've written it.

## What is Your Motive?

There may be many reasons that you are reading this book. Perhaps you have osteopenia or osteoporosis, or just want to strengthen and build your bones. You may have a parent, relative, or friend that needs your help to improve their bone health. Maybe you are a healthcare professional looking for a book that incorporates exercises that you can recommend to your patients and those to which you provide care.

Your goals may include things, such as

- ✧ better balance, coordination, and stability
- ✧ building and maintaining bone density
- ✧ developing better posture and body alignment
- ✧ gaining and keeping strength to accomplish everyday activities
- ✧ increasing flexibility and mobility
- ✧ improving cardiovascular and overall physical fitness
- ✧ preventing falls and fractures
- ✧ reducing bone loss

This book offers some basic information about bone health and 60 osteoporosis-friendly exercises to help build better bones.

# My Personal Connection

Just like you have a motive for reading this book, I have one for writing it. The many side effects of osteoporosis touched someone that is dear to me. Here is her story.

"Her eyes were smiling but her body was in pain. She wanted to play golf, jump into a pile of leaves, or go roller skating with her students like she used to do when she was younger. But her bones were porous and brittle, full of tiny holes. The doctor called it osteoporosis. All she knew was that she was in chronic pain and her joints were stiff. Because of the constant wear of discomfort all day every day, she found herself no longer able to work at the school. She sat at home most days hoping that someone would come by to visit but very few people did."

I met my favorite teacher when I was in high school. Being a teenager, I didn't really want to be in English class and I certainly didn't want to write a three-paragraph essay about the book I was supposed to have read. But Mrs. Griffith was a different kind of teacher. She didn't threaten or nag me when I turned in sub-par work week after week. Instead, she was funny, kind, and filled with grace. Mrs. Griffith loved her students, loved teaching, and it showed. She encouraged me to finish high school and look forward to a future of doing something I loved. So I did both.

Once I had graduated, I moved away from my hometown to pursue my goals. But whenever I came back home to visit, I would always stop by and see Mrs. Griffith at the high school. She would share with me stories about her "special students" that were a lot like I was. We'd laugh and reminisce about my year in her class. I appreciated that she would ask me what I was doing currently and tell me how proud she was of how far I had come.

Several years later, I went back to my hometown again and stopped in to see my former teacher but found she was no longer working at the school. She had had some health problems, they told me, so she retired. I went to visit her at her home and was saddened to learn that Mrs. Griffith

had developed osteoporosis. She had fallen and broken her hip. It was healing but was giving her a great deal of pain. Osteoporosis caused her to struggle in her daily activities and overall ability to enjoy certain things in life. It grieved me to see my former teacher, who was once so active, in this condition.

After seeing the real effects of osteoporosis on a person that is important to me, I wanted to put together an exercise book that addressed this issue. In addition to good nutrition and good health habits, exercise is an important key to good bone density.

But first, let's learn the information and statistics about bone health and osteoporosis.

# What is Osteoporosis?

Your bones are amazing. They are living tissue in your body that replenishes themselves continually. Similar to your blood, hair, fingernail, and skin cells, your bone cells are constantly growing and replacing the old with the new. Just think, because of this, you have a brand new skeleton about every ten years!

Osteoclasts and osteoblasts are the bone cells responsible for the ongoing renewal of your bones. They work in conjunction with each other to clear away old bone and replace it with new bone tissue. As we age, however, osteoblasts have a harder time keeping up and replacing new tissue with the old tissue that is being removed.

Osteoporosis is a bone disease. It comes from Greek and Latin as many medical terms do. "Osteo" means bone, "por" means small opening or passageway, and "osis" means a pathological condition. Together, these words mean "porous bone condition." Osteopenia is less severe than osteoporosis, but left untreated it can progress into osteoporosis.

Normally young and healthy bone tissue is hard on the outside and spongy on the inside. The inside spongy tissue is packed densely full of microscopic holes. When a person has osteopenia or osteoporosis, this spongy tissue becomes less dense and develops larger holes. These larger holes weaken the structure of the bone and cause it to become more brittle. The three areas of the body where weakened bones are vulnerable to fractures and breaks are the hip, spine, and wrists.

## Who is Affected

While anyone can develop osteoporosis, there are certain populations that are affected more prevalently. According to the National Library of Medicine , you are at higher risk for developing a bone disease if you have certain characteristics (Porter & Varacallo, 2019):

✧ **Alcoholism:** The continued use of heavy alcohol drinking contributes to the loss of bone density.

✧ **Corticosteroid user:** Those who take this class of medication are more susceptible.

✧ **Deficient in vitamin D:** The incidence of fractures is higher in those who are lacking adequate levels of this vitamin.

✧ **Female:** Between 9% and 38% of females are affected by osteoporosis versus 2% to 8% of males.

✧ **Genetically predisposed:** Those with a family history of osteoporosis are more likely to develop it.

✧ **Lower in body weight:** Those weighing less than 128 pounds are more likely to be affected.

✧ **Over 80 years old:** More than 70% of the elderly population is affected.

✧ **Physically inactive:** People with low levels of exercise and activity are more likely to be affected.

✧ **A smoker:** People who smoke are more susceptible to developing osteoporosis.

✧ **White or Asian:** The incidence of osteoporosis is higher in these races.

## What are the Complications

How do osteopenia and osteoporosis affect the quality of your daily life? Because of brittle or weakened bones, people with this condition can suffer a variety of consequences. According to the Office of the Surgeon General , some of these may include (National Library of Medicine, 2019):

✧ **anxiety and depression:** Anxiousness about falling and depression about the inability to safely participate in some activities rises for those with bone disease.

✧ **financial expenses:** Having a bone disease can be expensive. Some costs and drug therapy may not be covered by a person's insurance or Medicare. Many times these additional costs, especially ones associated with recovering from a broken bone, come out of the patient's pocket.

✧ **greater risk of breaks and fractures:** As we age, our balance and response reflex decrease making us more susceptible to falls. For those with brittle bones, these falls are more likely to cause a break or fracture. Suffering from a serious fracture in a major bone like the hip can start a spiral downward in health and well-being.

✧ **increased pain:** Falls and fractures resulting from bone disease can cause significant pain and impaired movement. One in five people who experience multiple fractures or a debilitating one will wind up in a nursing home because of their inability to stand, walk, or care for their daily needs.

✧ **limited activities:** Those with a bone disease should avoid certain activities that are jarring, jerking, twisting, and are accompanied by a higher risk of falling. Sports that involve moves like this are downhill skiing, golf, high-impact aerobics, ice skating, horseback riding, roller skating, and tennis.

✧ **loss of height:** Brittle bones can cause a collapse in the spinal vertebrae leading to a hunched-over spine, loss in height, and pain.

# Actions You Can Take

As we have discovered, there are certain things you cannot control in regard to your risk factors for developing osteopenia or osteoporosis. These factors include age, body size and stature, ethnicity, gender (according to chromosomes at birth, not by personal choice or surgery), and genetics. Fortunately or unfortunately, these are the cards that we all have been dealt in life.

The good news is there are many risk factors over which you have complete control. These components include alcohol consumption, medication choices, nutrient-rich food (with enough calcium and vitamin D), regular exercise, and smoking. These lifestyle changes are simple enough but require determination and planning to achieve.

This book is focused on the exercise component. We all know that regular physical activity is important for anyone who wants to maintain good health, but it is especially key for those with osteoporosis. However, we do want to talk briefly about the role of nutrition.

## *The Importance of Good Foods*

We all like to eat, don't we? Everyone has a favorite meal, special dessert, or irresistible snack that they love. These are all fine to indulge in from time to time, but our daily eating habits determine our health. For those with a bone disease, nutrition can play an important key in preventing further bone loss and boosting general well-being. According to a recent study, a healthy diet is important to the integrity of the bones and the reduction of fractures. The key nutrients needed are calcium, protein, and vitamin D. But magnesium, phosphorous, vitamin K, and zinc have also been shown to be important, too (Higgs et al., 2017).

So, what does an osteoporosis-friendly diet look like? The Mayo Clinic recommends (Weiss, 2022):

- **calcium:** Examples include dairy products, like cheese, milk, and yogurt, plant-based milks, like almond, cashew, and oat, and vegetables high in calcium, such as broccoli and kale.
- **fruits, vegetables, and grains:** A variety of fruits and vegetables provide vitamins A, C, and K as well as phytonutrients and minerals. Whole grains are a good source of fiber and magnesium.
- **protein and fat:** Examples are chicken, fish, lean meats, and other animal protein sources, while plant protein includes beans, nuts, and seeds. Protein should be 25% to 35% of the calories you take in each day.
- **vitamin D:** It's called the sunshine vitamin because exposure to sunlight helps your body produce it naturally. It can also be found in eggs, fish and seafood, and mushrooms.
- **limit alcohol, caffeine, salt, and sugar:** You may be thinking "well, there goes all the fun," but these can be enjoyed in moderation. Just not every day.

## *The Importance of Exercise*

Exercise is essential for everyone. If you want to prevent or help treat bone disease, exercising is a crucial element in achieving that goal. How does exercise do that?

When we regularly move our bodies, train our muscles, and exercise our cardiovascular system, it is like making a deposit into our good health account. Exercise helps us improve our balance, flexibility, posture, and muscle strength as well as our heart health. When all these things are made stronger, we enjoy better health physically, mentally, and even financially by avoiding trips to the doctor.

Because bones are living and growing tissue, they become stronger when you exercise. Resistance training and weight-bearing exercises are best for those who want to better their bone health. Both of these types of exercise use resistance against gravity or your own body weight. This resistance applies pressure to the skeleton causing the osteoblasts (remember those?) to create new bone tissue.

Some common osteoporosis-friendly exercise examples include the following.

### Resistance Training

- free weights (ankle weights, dumbbells, kettlebells, medicine balls, water bottles, weighted vests)
- machine weights (cables, hamstring extension, quad extension, plus others)
- pilates
- resistance bands

✧ yoga

**Weight-Bearing Exercises**

✧ dancing

✧ elliptical

✧ hiking

✧ low-impact aerobics

✧ stair climbing

✧ walking

Weight-bearing exercises are also considered impact-loading. What does this mean? Impact-loading exercises require contact with the ground or a stationary object. These exercises can be low-impact, moderate-impact, or high-impact. Those with weakened bones should stick to low-impact to moderate-impact exercises. A recent study has shown that impact-loading exercises can substantially increase bone density (Sundh et al., 2018).

One of the ways that weight-bearing exercises—such as dancing and low-impact aerobics—are especially good for bone building is because they also incorporate what is called "odd-impact" loading. In some trial studies, it was shown that odd-impact loading exercises can contribute to higher bone density as much as high-impact ones do (Gulbrandson, 2019). The reason given for the success of odd-impact loading exercises is that these provide a type of movement that surprises your bones. They require your muscles to move in different ways and pull at your bones at odd angles. Think about dancing, for instance. You are moving forward and backward, to the side and at an angle, with small steps and big steps, swooping and turning. Your muscles and your bones are constantly challenged and surprised by your movements. It's one more reason to add variety to your exercise routine!

## *Making a Decision*

Making a decision requires you to progress through a series of steps.

1. Pinpoint a goal. What do you want to achieve? What is important to you?
2. Educate yourself. Learn the needed information

to make a wise choice about what to do and how to get there.
3. Think about the alternatives and consequences. What are your other options? And what will happen if you don't make the decision?
4. Make the decision! And follow it with action. From there, you can evaluate if it is getting you closer toward your goal.

Now that you have determined your motive, learned about osteoporosis and its effects, identified your risk factors, and educated yourself on the benefits of exercise, it is time to make a decision. What are you going to do with the information you have?

Stronger bones don't just happen. Action on your part is required and that is preceded by a decision. You are in charge of your body, your choices, your mind, and your health. Perhaps you are worried about your current lack of physical fitness, the recent weight you have put on, or your non-athletic past. Maybe some of you were once superstar athletes and are discouraged that you aren't able to do what you used to. Listen, no one can compete with their 20-year-old selves. The past failures or successes in your life don't matter at this point!

Consider the alternative. If you do nothing, then nothing will change. Your bones will slowly weaken and your health will deteriorate. By making a decision today to improve your physical well-being, you are taking a step into your future self. That self is strong, healthy, and getting better all the time.

We encourage you to continue on your journey to better bone health by implementing the exercise plan outlined in this book. Let's take a look at what is included in the following chapters.

# How to Use This Book

Before starting any type of exercise program, please check in with your doctor or healthcare provider. Each person and their health history is different. We respect these differences and any modifications that your doctor may make regarding the exercises we have outlined. Some of the exercises in the next few chapters might not be a good fit for you and your current level of physical fitness or bone health. Consult with your healthcare provider and follow their recommendations for your specific situation.

The book is arranged into three major sections: Part 1, Part 2, and Part 3.

## *Part 1: The Foundation*

You've just finished reading Part 1 (congratulations!) where we talked about your motive, how this book came about, information about osteoporosis (including who is at risk and what the complications are), and actions you can take (including the importance of exercise and making a decision). Now you have a good foundation for understanding what is coming in Parts 2 and 3.

## *Part 2: The Exercises*

Part 2 consists of exercises that will help improve specific body functions. The exercises are grouped by chapter into targeted areas. Each of these chapters features exercises that will help you improve on a certain skill, such as balance, flexibility, posture, strength, and cardio. Remember that you may need to make modifications to some exercises to accommodate your individual fitness level and ability.

Included with each exercise is the following information:

1) Time needed to perform it.
2) Directions on how it is done.
3) Web link to view either pictures or a video that shows proper form.
4) How to level up or make it more challenging.
5) Cautions on what not to do.
6) How the exercise benefits you and what part of the body it is targeting.

The chapters include:

- ✧ **Chapter 1: Improving Your Balance:** Our ability to balance and remain stable while performing everyday tasks can decrease over

time. However, a loss of balance can put you at risk of falling, tripping, and potentially breaking or fracturing bones. But balance can be improved! These twelve exercises focus on enhancing your balance and stability. No equipment is needed.

- ✧ **Chapter 2: Improving Your Flexibility:** It's not just about being able to touch your toes. Flexibility is needed for daily living. A decrease in flexibility can cause muscle tightness, back pain, and a higher chance of injury. The exercises outlined in this chapter will help you become looser, stretchier, and maintain a full range of motion in your joints. No equipment is needed.

- ✧ **Chapter 3: Improving Your Posture:** Beauty and pageant queens understand it: good posture gives you confidence while also protecting your back and spine. Practicing good posture also helps you breathe better and alleviate back pain. The twelve exercises in this chapter guide you toward proper posture and alignment. No equipment is needed.

- ✧ **Chapter 4: Improving Your Strength:** Muscle mass starts to decline after age 30, so it is important to work on building it back. When muscles decrease or lose strength, it puts us at a greater risk for disability and falls. Preserving muscle strength ensures that we will be strong enough to not only accomplish our necessary activities but also enjoy life. The exercises in this chapter are designed to build the strength in your arm, leg, and core muscles. It is helpful to have a few pieces of equipment for the strength exercises but they are easily found around your home.

- ✧ **Chapter 5: Improving Your Cardio:** Good heart and circulatory health keep us active and engaged with family and friends. Regular cardio exercise helps our bodies to fight off illness, keep extra weight off, increase our stamina, and boost our mood. Included are some common and some not-so-common cardio exercises that are weight-bearing, osteoporosis-friendly, and fun. Some of the cardio exercises require equipment that is found at the gym or can be purchased for home use. Variety is important for any type of exercise, but especially for cardio. It keeps our minds and muscles from getting bored.

## Part 3: The Action Plan

Here is where we put it all together! Looking at five chapters of exercises can get overwhelming. What to do first? How to combine training and cardio? We have made it easy for you by assembling exercise routines in Chapter 6. Included is a month's worth of exercise routines, broken down by weeks. The routines are for five days of exercise and two days of rest. You get to choose your rest days to accommodate your schedule. Going away for the weekend? Take those two days as your rest days. You can mix and match the days to fit your needs.

Each week features a 3-2 combo of resistance training and weight-bearing cardio. Some weeks will have three days of cardio and the following week will have two. The cardio days are alternated with training days. This ensures that you aren't doing the same thing every day and every week. Remember, your muscles need to be surprised!

**Week 1:** The program this week will consist of days one, three, and five being resistance training. Days two and four will be cardio. Cardio is kept to 20 minutes or less.

**Week 2:** This week will have you do cardio on days one, three, and five. Resistance training will be performed on days two and four. This is where you start to gain momentum and consistency.

**Week 3:** You are building stamina now! Days one, three,

and five feature resistance training. Cardio will be on days two and four. Cardio goes a few minutes longer this week.

**Week 4:** This week, the cardio is on days one, three, and five. Days two and four are for resistance training. Cardio is upped slightly again this week as you get stronger.

## Hope

Are you feeling hopeful? I am. There is real change ahead for you. It is my hope that you are excited to embark on this amazing journey to build stronger bones and enjoy the benefits of better bone health. There is some hard work ahead of you, but you can do it and I will show you how.

Let's get started.

# Part 2:
# The Exercises

*Exercise to stimulate, not to annihilate. The world wasn't formed in a day, and neither were we. Set small goals and build upon them.*

**Lee Haney**

# Chapter 1
# Improving Your Balance

D id you walk across the room today? Or stand up from a chair? How about turning your head to look at something behind you? We use our balance for just about everything in our average day-to-day living.

As we age, our balance can become a challenge because of the many changes that happen in our bodies.

> Step with care and great tact, and remember that Life's a Great Balancing Act.
>
> *Dr. Seuss*

Some balance issues are related to blood pressure, medication, and vestibular or other neurological problems. Having good balance helps to avoid falls and trips that could result in breaks and fractures, particularly for those with brittle or porous bones.

In this chapter, we will be improving your balance through 12 exercises that will build your ability to remain stable while doing everyday activities. No equipment is needed for these; but have a sturdy chair and mat available.

# BALANCE EXERCISES

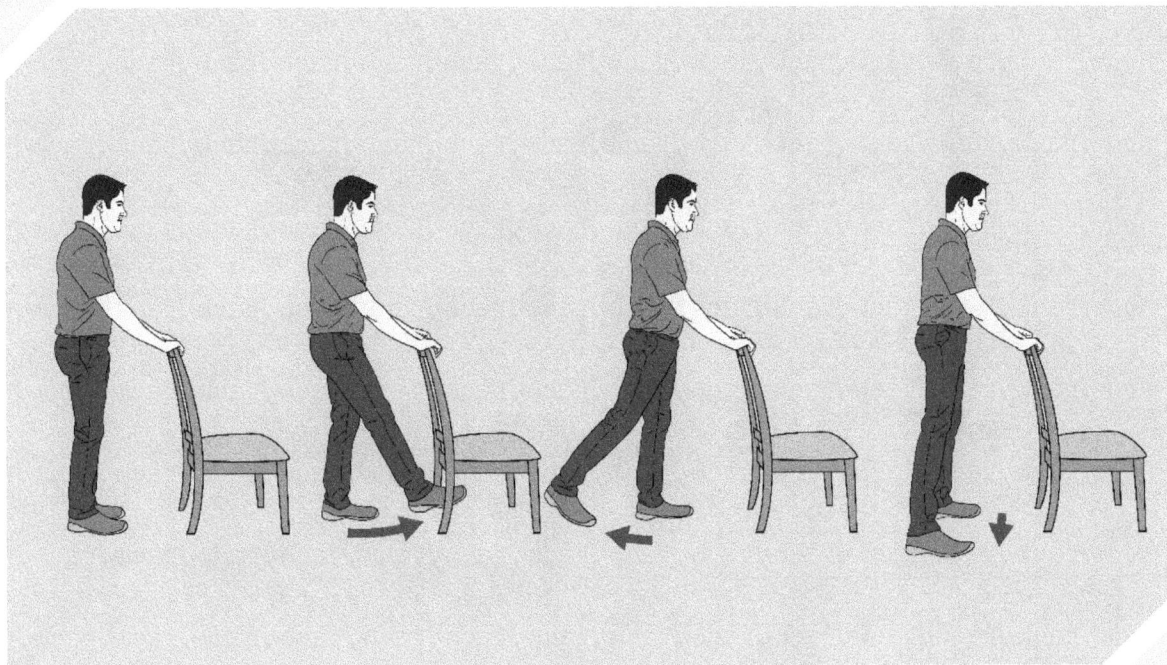

# 3 WAY HIP KICK

## Time Needed: Three minutes

## Directions:

1. Stand up straight with your feet apart and directly below your hips. Use your hand for support by placing it on a sturdy chair, countertop, or wall for support.

2. Extend your right foot forward in front of you. Return your foot back to where it was at the starting position.

3. Extend your right foot to the right side and then back to the starting position.

4. Now, reach your right foot back behind you, then back to the starting position.

5. Repeat with the right foot a total of five times.

6. Switch to the left foot and repeat the cycle of front, side, and back five times on the left.

7. Do the exercise again two more times on each side.

**Cautions:** Do not lean forward or backward while performing this exercise. Your leg is the only thing that should be moving here. Your body should remain upright.

**Level Up:** Do this exercise without holding onto anything for support. Place your hands on your hips for added balance.

**Benefits:** Helps with balance and stability by strengthening hip muscles and increasing mobility.

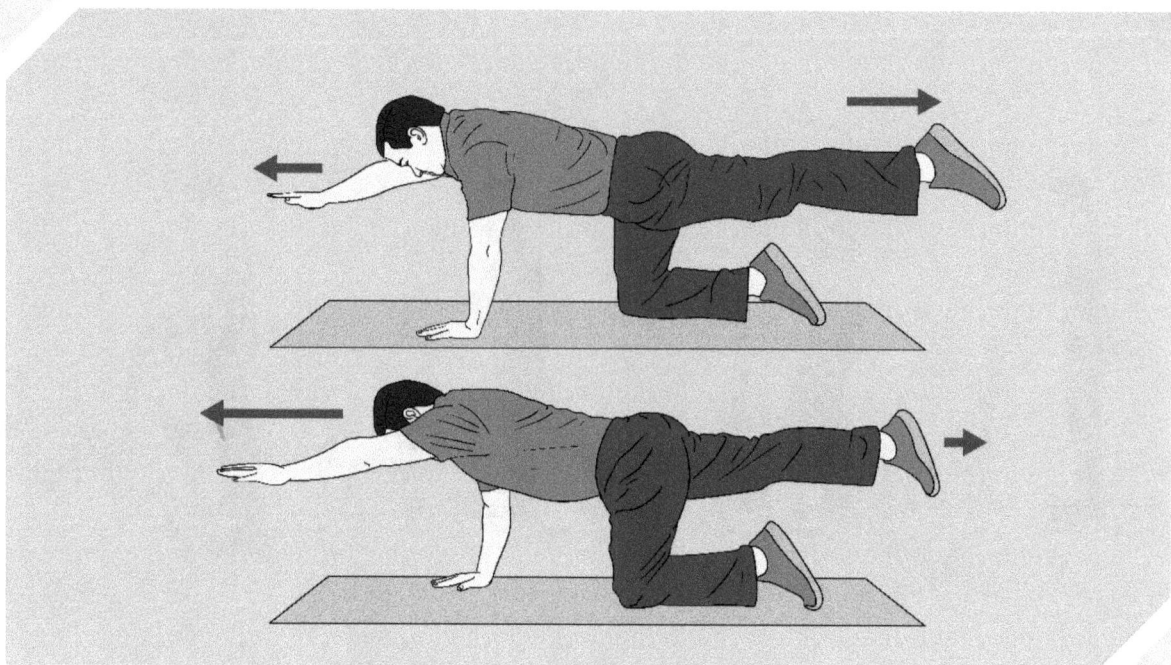

# Bird Dog

## Time Needed: Three minutes

## Directions:

1.  Get down on the floor or a padded mat on your knees and hands, with your knees directly under your hips and hands directly under your shoulders. Keep your back in a neutral position and look down towards the floor or slightly forward.

2.  Engage your core as you extend your right arm in front of you and extend your left leg behind you, lifting both until they are parallel to the ground. Slowly lower your arm and leg back down to starting position.

3.  Repeat the movement on the opposite side by extending your left arm in front of you and your right leg behind you, then lower back down. This is one rep.

4.  Repeat and perform eight reps in total.

**Cautions:** Don't arch your back or let it sag when you perform this, just keep your spine neutral.

**Level Up:** To make this harder, pause and hold your arm and leg in the lifted position for five seconds before lowering to the ground.

**Benefits:** Core muscles are important for overall balance and this exercise will strengthen them.

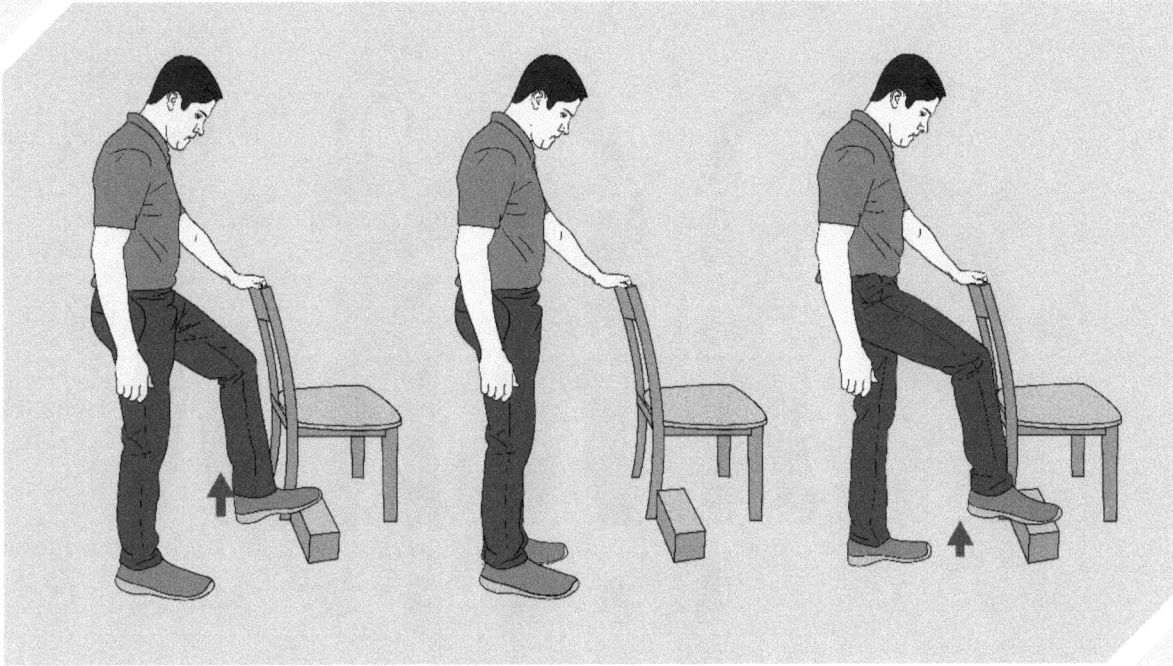

# FOOT TAPS

## Time Needed: Three minutes

## Directions:

1. Stand up straight holding onto a wall or countertop for support. Have a yoga block on its highest side or a small cone in front of you on the floor.

2. Lift your right foot and tap the top of the block or cone with your foot. Bring the foot back to the starting position. Repeat 10 times on this leg.

3. Switch legs and now lift your left foot and do the same lifting and tapping 10 times on the left leg. This is one set.

4. Repeat the set two more times.

**Cautions:** Lift your foot high enough to touch the top of the cone but do not lean forward or backward. Move with control and consistency.

**Level Up:** Make this more challenging by not holding onto anything for support and putting your hands on your hips.

**An extra challenge:** alternate feet each time.

**Benefits:** Helps improve balance and coordination on stair steps to avoid trips and falls.

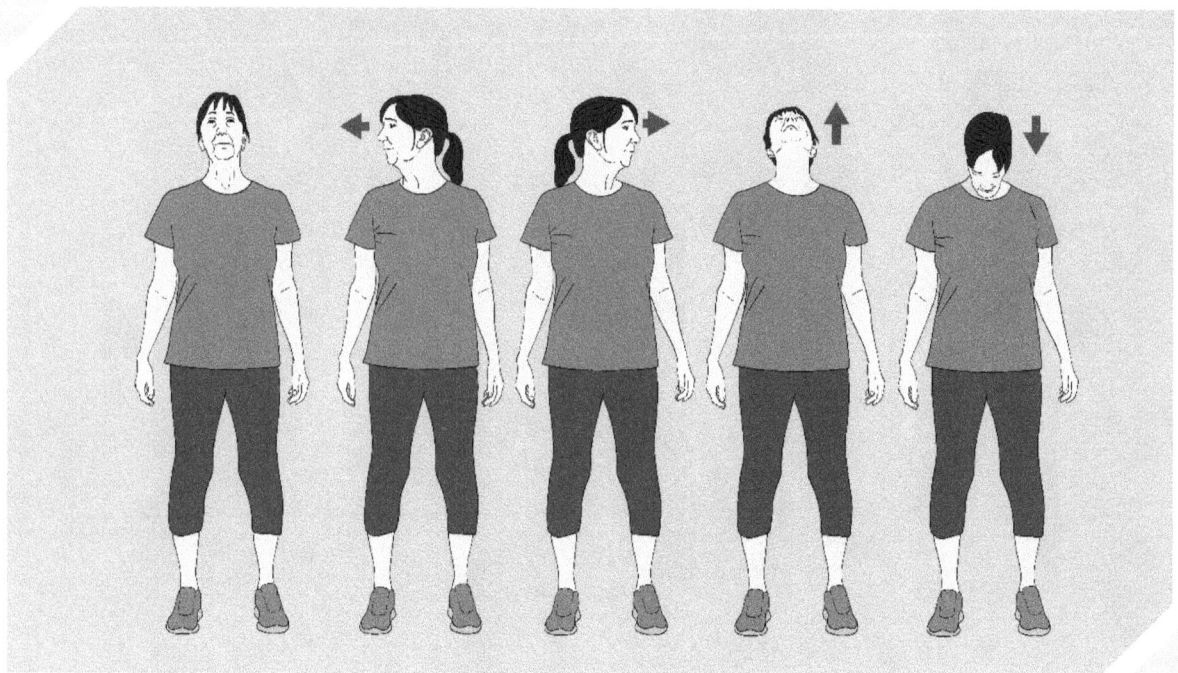

# HEAD ROTATION

## Time Needed: One minute

## Directions:

1.  Stand up straight with your feet a hip-width distance apart. Have one hand on a countertop or sturdy chair for support.

2.  Keeping your body still, move your head to look to the right and then the left. Now move it to look up and look down. Repeat several times for 30 seconds.

3.  Rest, then do it again for another 30 seconds.

**Cautions:** This may cause dizziness. If you feel dizzy, stop immediately. Rest, then try it again more slowly.

**Level Up:** Make this more challenging by not holding onto anything for support.

**Benefits:** Helps to engage the brain and body connection for better balance while increasing mobility in the neck.

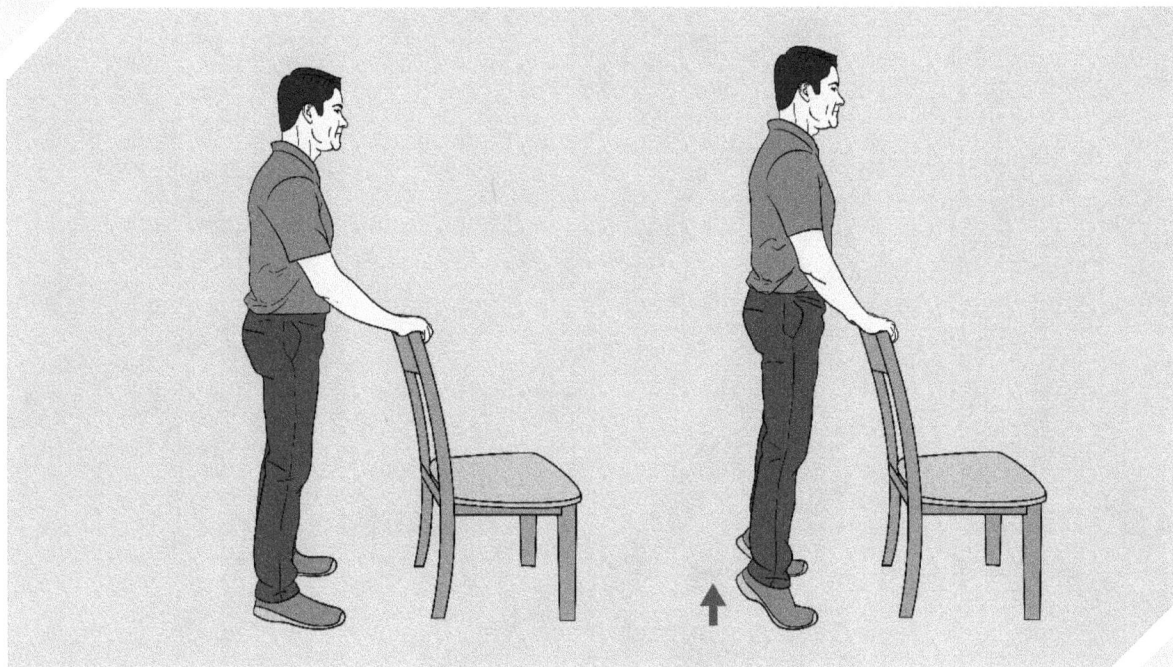

# HEEL RAISES

## Time Needed: Two minutes

### Directions:

1. With feet hip-width apart, stand erect. If you need support, lay both hands on a countertop or sturdy chair.

2. Raise up both heels off the ground simultaneously. Don't lean forward. Keep your posture and head erect. Lower your heels back down to the floor.

3. Repeat the heel raises for a total of 10 times. This is one set.

4. Perform three more sets.

**Cautions:** Watch for cramping in your calf muscles, especially if you are performing these for the first time. Rest until the cramp goes away and try again.

**Level Up:** As you get stronger, only use one hand for support, then no hands.

**Benefits:** Strengthens calf and ankle muscles, which adds to overall balance and support in the lower body.

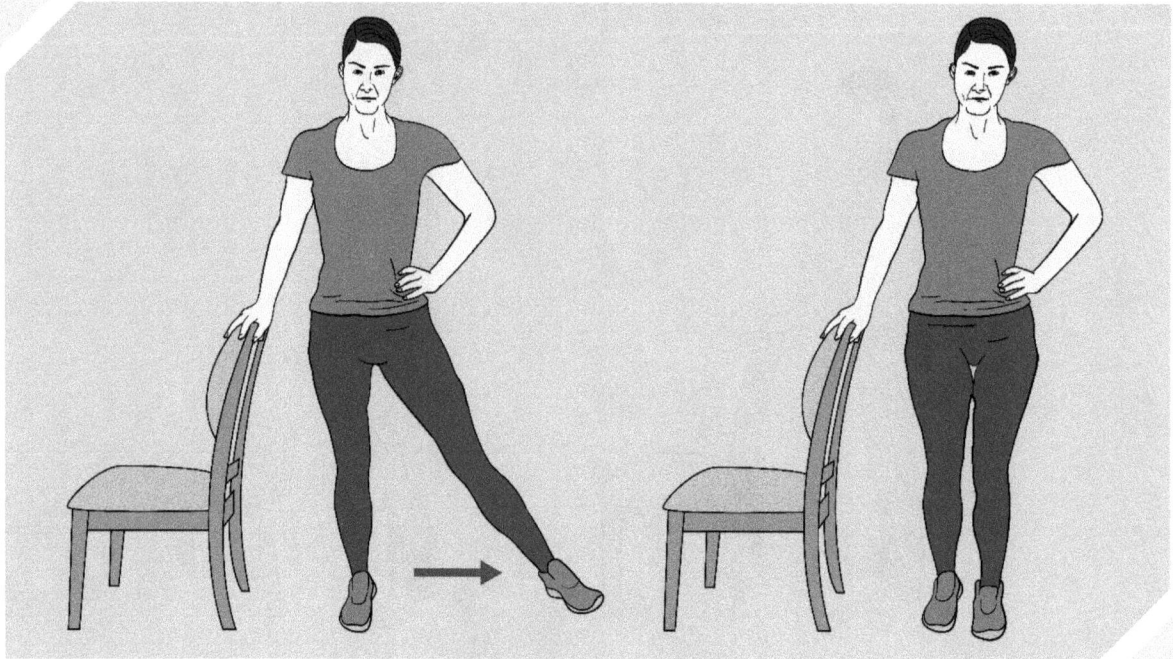

# HIP ABDUCTOR

---

**Time Needed:** Three minutes

---

## Directions:

1. Stand up straight next to a counter or sturdy chair and put your left hand on it for support. Take your right hand and place it on your hip.

2. Raise your right leg in a straight line out to the right side. Return it to the floor. Repeat for a total of 10 times.

3. Switch sides by putting your right hand on the counter and your left hand on your hip. Lift your left leg to the side 10 times. This is one set.

4. Repeat for two more sets.

**Cautions:** Keep your toes pointed forward as you lift and don't lean to either side as it may throw you off balance.

**Level Up:** Make this more challenging by adding ankle weights.

**Benefits:** Brings balance and stability by strengthening the hip muscles.

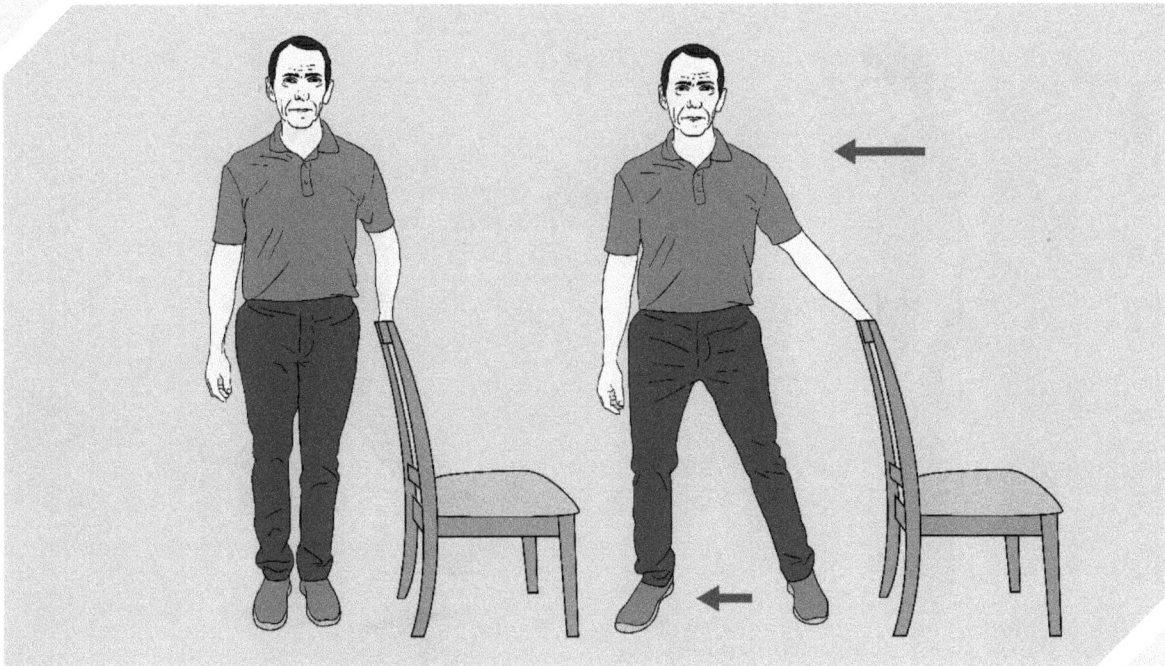

# LATERAL STEPPING

## Time Needed: Three minutes

## Directions:

1. Stand up straight with your feet together. Hold on to a countertop or railing for support.

2. Using your right foot step sideways to the right in a normal-sized step. Continue stepping to the right for 10 steps total.

3. Now, use your left foot to step sideways to the left for 10 steps. This is one set.

4. Repeat stepping for two more sets.

**Cautions:** Don't make your steps too big as it may cause you to feel off-balance. Ensure that there are no potential tripping hazards in your exercise path.

**Level Up:** Make this more challenging by crossing your foot in front or behind your other foot as you step. For example, use your left foot to step to the right by crossing in front of your right foot. Then step with your right foot to continue moving to the right.

**Benefits:** Builds balance and coordination, especially when stepping sideways to get out of someone's way or turning around in crowded spaces.

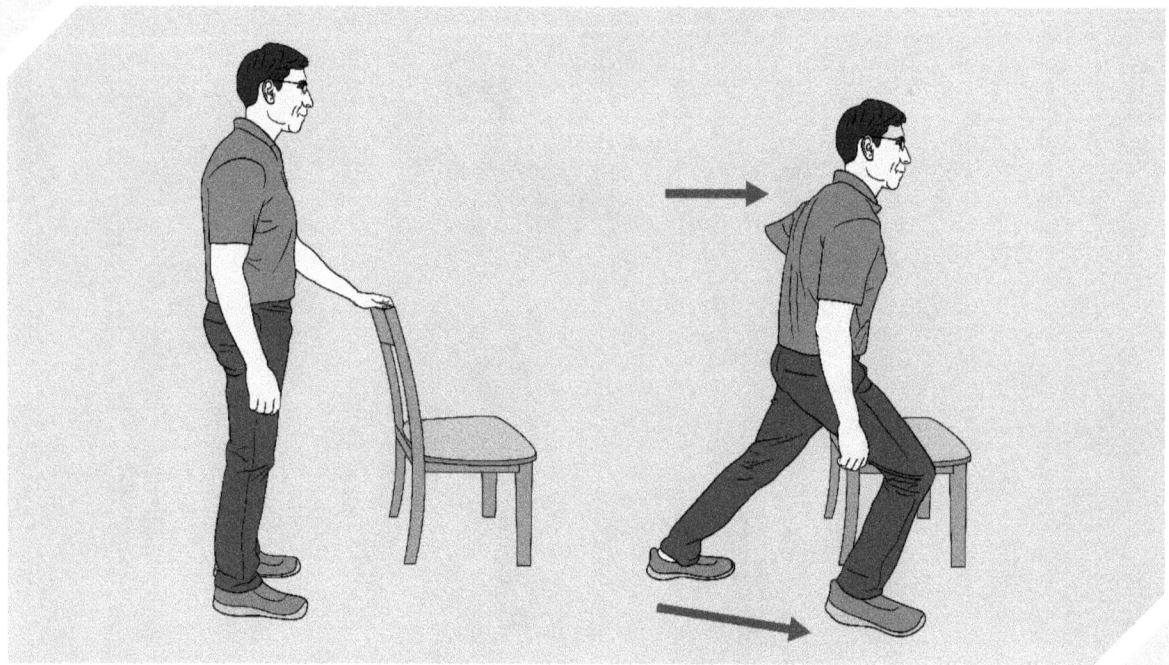

# MINI-LUNGE

## Time Needed: Five minutes

## Directions:

1. Stand up straight with your feet hip-width apart. Place your hand on a counter or sturdy chair for support.

2. Step your right foot forward and bend your right knee in a mini-lunge. It does not need to be too deep. Return your foot to the starting position. Repeat for a total of 10 lunges on this leg.

3. Switch legs and step your left foot forward and bend your left knee in a mini-lunge for a total of 10 times. This is one set.

4. Repeat for two more sets.

**Cautions:** Resist the urge to do these quickly. It's better to perform controlled and consistent lunges.

**Level Up:** Instead of using a counter for support, place your hands on your hips while performing the lunges for an extra challenge.

**Benefits:** Helps with balance and stability while stepping forward with a change in center of gravity.

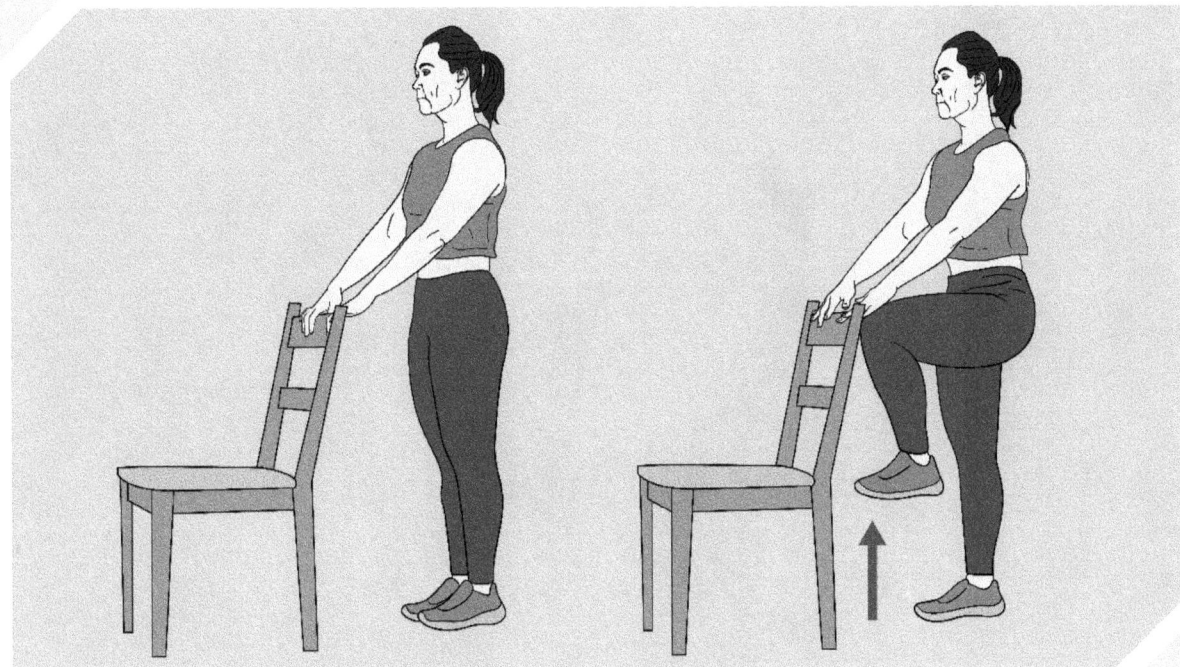

# SINGLE LEG STANCE

**Time Needed:** Five minutes

## Directions:

1. Stand near a counter or sturdy chair and place one hand on it for support. Your feet should be hip-width apart.

2. Lift the right foot off the ground with your knee slightly bent in front of you and hold it up for 10 seconds. Return the foot to the starting position. Repeat for a total of five times on this leg.

3. Repeat the exercise on the left leg a total of five times. This completes one set.

4. Do the set once more on each leg.

**Cautions:** Don't lean over or put added pressure on the foot that is on the ground. Remain standing straight up while doing the exercise.

**Level Up:** Make this more challenging by not holding onto anything for support and having your hands on your hips. You can also hold your foot up for 15 or 20 seconds.

**Benefits:** Builds balance and stamina for walking, going up and down stairs, and getting out of cars.

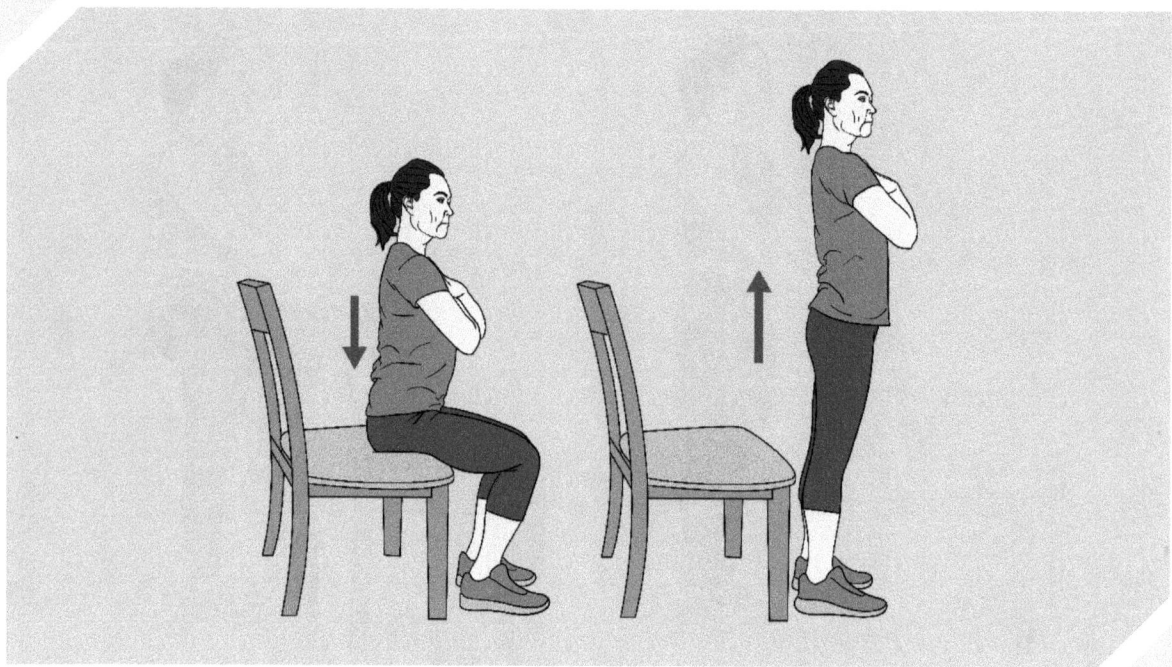

# SIT TO STAND

**Time Needed:** Three minutes

## Directions:

1. Sit erect in a sturdy chair with both feet on the ground and knees bent. Place your arms criss-cross in front of you with your hands on your shoulders or behind your head.

2. Engage your core and leg muscles as you rise up to a straight-up standing position. Slowly lower back down to the seated starting position.

3. Repeat the move a total of 10 times. This is one set.

4. Perform the set two more times.

**Cautions:** Be sure the chair you are using does not have wheels on the bottom. If you don't feel stable yet doing this without the use of your hands, let your hands help you lift off the chair.

**Level Up:** Increase the difficulty by adding hand weights.

**Benefits:** Helps with balance and mobility in the hips and back to perform everyday activities.

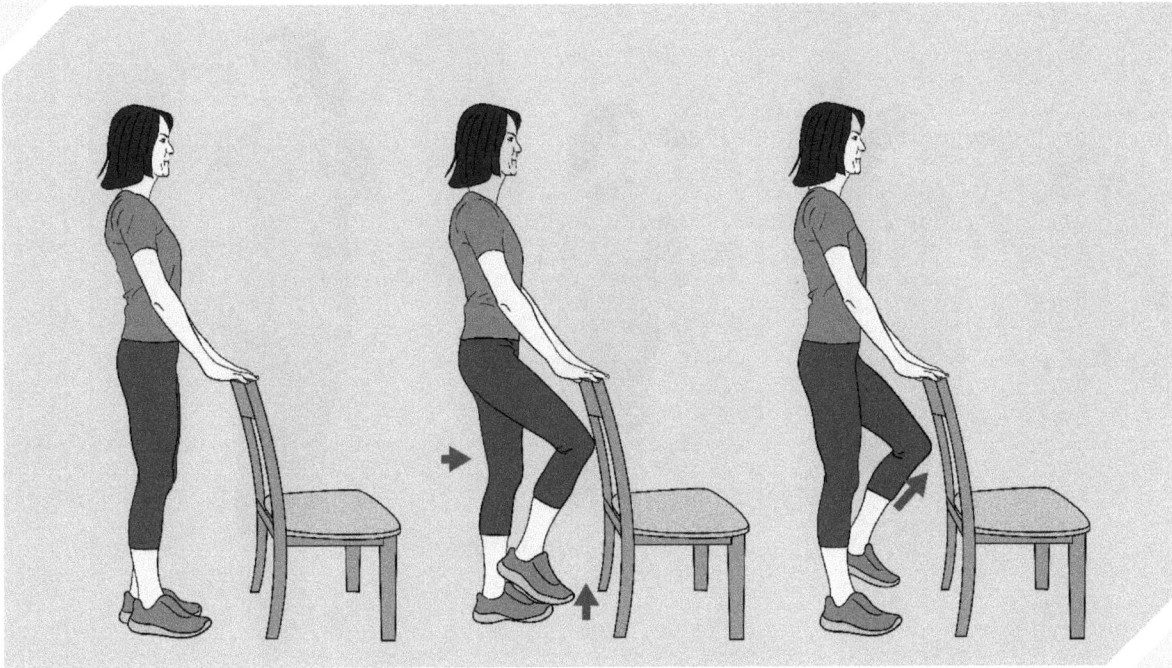

# STANDING MARCHES

**Time Needed:** Two minutes

## Directions:

1. Stand up straight with one hand on a countertop or sturdy chair.

2. Bend and lift your right leg until your knee is almost the same height as your hip. Bring the foot back down to the starting position.

3. Switch legs and do the same on your left leg, as if you were marching.

4. Repeat marching 10 times on each leg. This is one set.

5. Perform three more sets.

**Cautions:** Don't lean to the right or the left as you march. Keep your body erect and tall.

**Level Up:** Make this more difficult by not holding onto anything and placing your hands on your hips.

**Benefits:** Improves balance by strengthening hips.

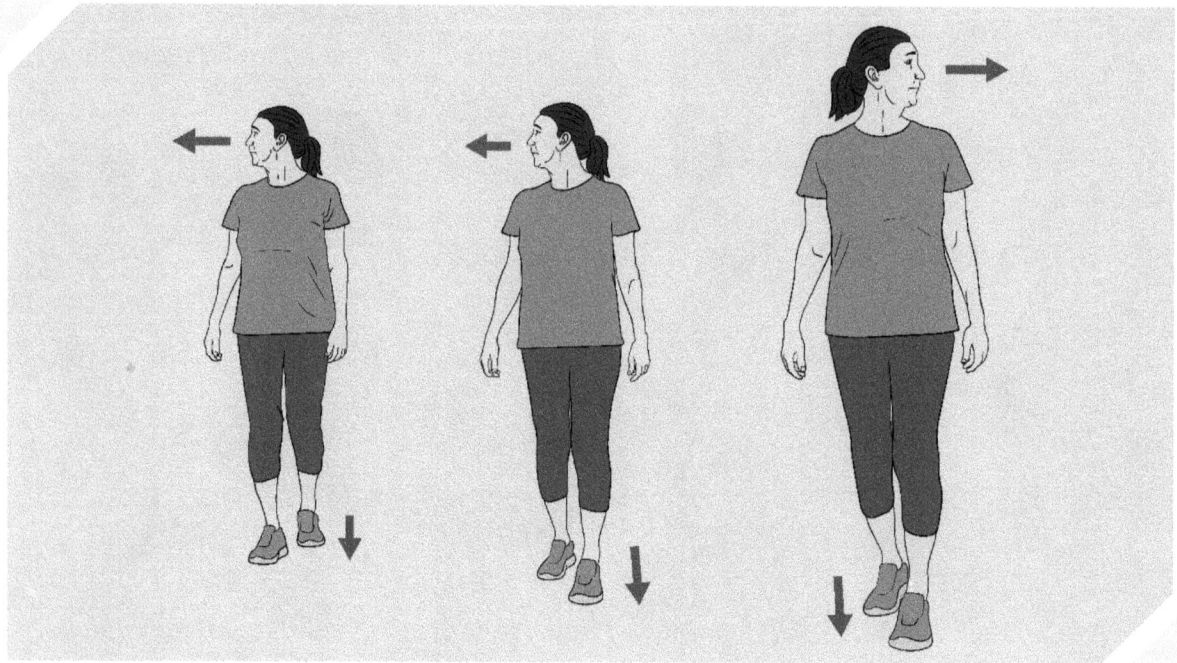

# OVER-THE-SHOULDER WALKS

## Time Needed: Two minutes

## Directions:

1. Stand at one end of the room or next to a long countertop. Hands can be down at your sides or one hand can be on the counter for support.

2. Look behind you to the right and walk five steps forward, then look to the left as you continue stepping forward five more steps. This is one set.

3. Repeat the set five more times.

**Cautions:** Have one hand on the wall or counter to prevent falls.

**Level Up:** As you progress, do this walk without holding onto anything for support.

**Benefits:** Helps to improve balance by engaging your brain and body to work together while walking.

# Chapter 2:
# Improving Your Flexibility

**W**hat comes to your mind when you hear the word flexible? Perhaps a gymnast doing the splits or an acrobat touching their nose to their knees? People who perform these moves are certainly flexible, but the average person is flexible, too. We all need a certain amount of flexibility to engage in normal

> " Flexibility is crucial to my fitness.
> **Samantha Stosur** "

everyday activities. Things like bending over to tie our shoes, getting in and out of vehicles, and reaching for something at the back of a shelf all require some measure of flexibility.

Our bodies get older and we lose some degree of elasticity in our tendons and muscles. The hips and shoulders are common areas to notice this loss. It is normal, but that doesn't mean we have to lose our ability to do simple activities because of flexibility problems. Good flexibility can lessen aches and pains, muscle strain, and the risk of falling.

In this chapter, we will improve your flexibility with twelve exercises that stretch your muscles in an osteoporosis-friendly way. No equipment is needed for these moves, but it is helpful to have a sturdy chair and padded mat available.

# FLEXIBILITY EXERCISES

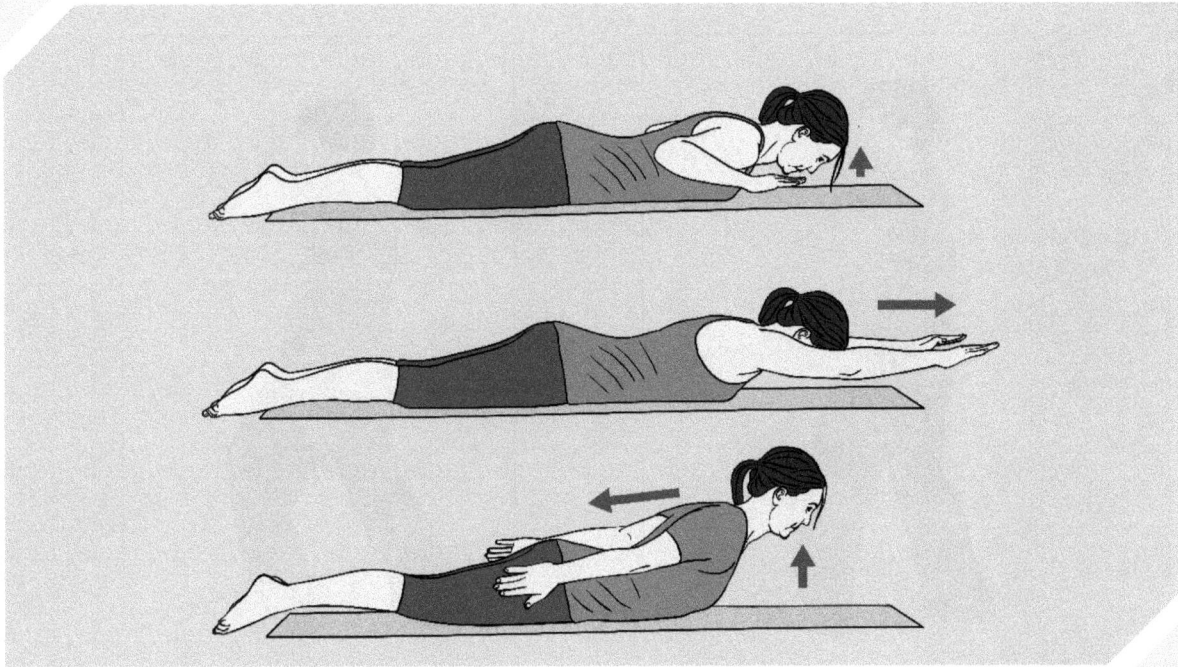

# BREASTSTROKE

**Time Needed:** Three minutes

## Directions:

1. Lie face down on the floor or on a padded mat. Legs are a hip-width distance apart and toes are pointed. Arms are bent at a 90-degree angle and in a cactus shape with palms facing down to the floor.

2. Inhale, then as you exhale reach your hands forward so they are in front of you, palms down. Your arms, torso, and legs should be in a straight line and your arms hovering above the mat.

3. Inhale again, then as you exhale, circle the arms out to the side and down to your sides with palms facing towards the sides of your body. Shoulders and upper ribs are hovering above the mat. Return to the starting position and rest for a few seconds.

4. Repeat the move a total of five times.

**Cautions:** Keep your shoulders relaxed and away from your ears to avoid scrunching up at the neck. Allow the neck to be long and lengthened.

**Level Up:** To increase the difficulty, don't pause between repeat movements. Make the move continuous and smooth.

**Benefits:** This keeps the muscles around your spine flexible and strengthened.

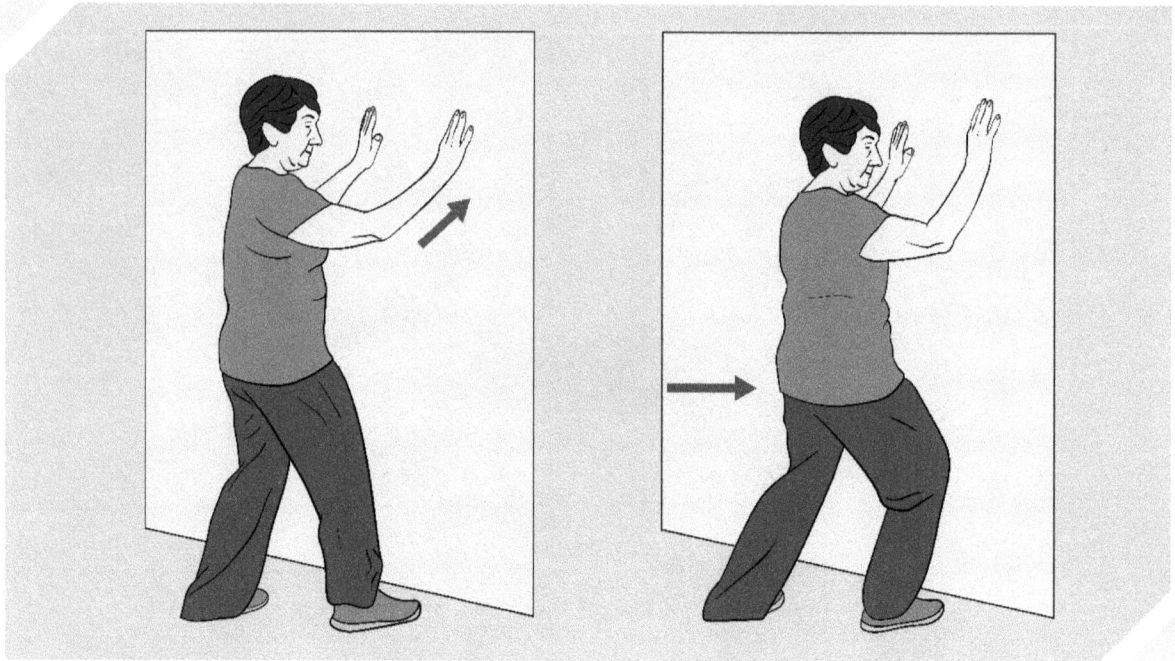

# CALF STRETCH

---

**Time Needed:** Two minutes

---

## Directions:

1.  Stand up straight facing a wall about an arms-length distance away. Your feet should be directly below your hip bones.

2.  Place your palms on the wall as you step your right foot to the wall while keeping your back leg straight. Keep your left leg straight while bending your right knee. You should feel a stretch in your left calf as you press into your left heel. Hold for 20 seconds then relax your legs. Do the stretch again on this leg.

3.  Switch legs by stepping forward with your left foot and keeping your right leg back and straight. Bend your left knee as you press into your right heel to stretch your right calf. Hold for 20 seconds then relax your legs. Do the stretch one more time on this leg.

**Cautions:** Take care not to hunch up your shoulders as you press your palms onto the wall. Keep your neck long and shoulders away from your ears.

**Level Up:** Hold the stretch a little longer for 30 or 45 seconds.

**Benefits:** Helps your calf to remain flexible and increases flexibility in your knee.

28

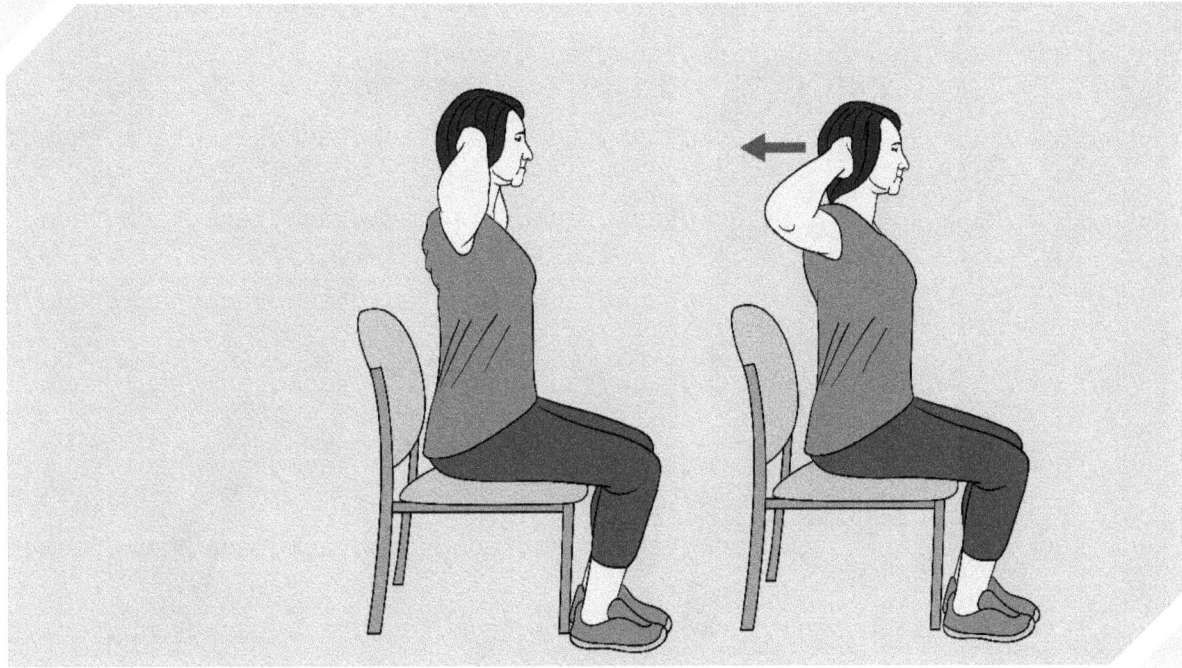

# CHEST STRETCH

**Time Needed:** One minute

## Directions:

1. Sit upright in a sturdy chair with feet flat on the floor and knees bent at a 90-degree angle.

2. Bend your arms at the elbow and place your hands behind your ears, head, or neck, depending on your shoulder mobility.

3. Take a deep breath in and slowly move both elbows backward until you feel a stretch in your chest and upper back. Exhale and allow elbows to come forward again.

4. Repeat the move four more times.

**Cautions:** Take care not to pull on your head or neck while moving elbows backward.

**Level Up:** Do this exercise while standing and you will be working on balance at the same time.

**Benefits:** Helps to stretch your chest and upper back increasing flexibility in these areas.

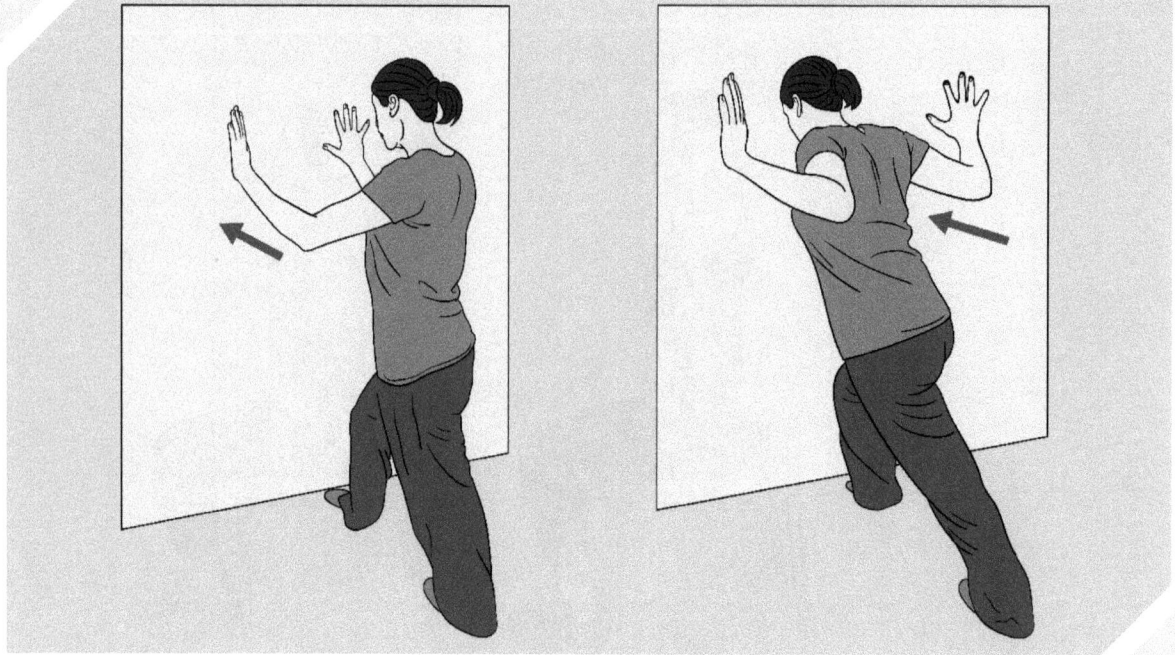

# CORNER STRETCH

## Time Needed: Four minutes

## Directions:

1. Find a corner of a room or other walls that meet at a 90-degree angle. Place arms in a cactus shape with upper arms in line with shoulders and hands up with palms on the walls.

2. Step forward with the right leg into the corner and lean onto it. Hold for 10 seconds. You should feel the stretch in the front of your shoulders. Return to the starting position.

3. Repeat the motion with the left leg by stepping forward into the corner and leaning onto it. This is one set.

4. Repeat for a total of five sets.

**Cautions:** Keep your shoulders pressed down and your neck long to avoid scrunching up.

**Level Up:** Hold the stretch in the corner for 20 to 30 seconds.

**Benefits:** Helps stretch the shoulders and opens up the chest. Counteracts rounded shoulders and hunching forward.

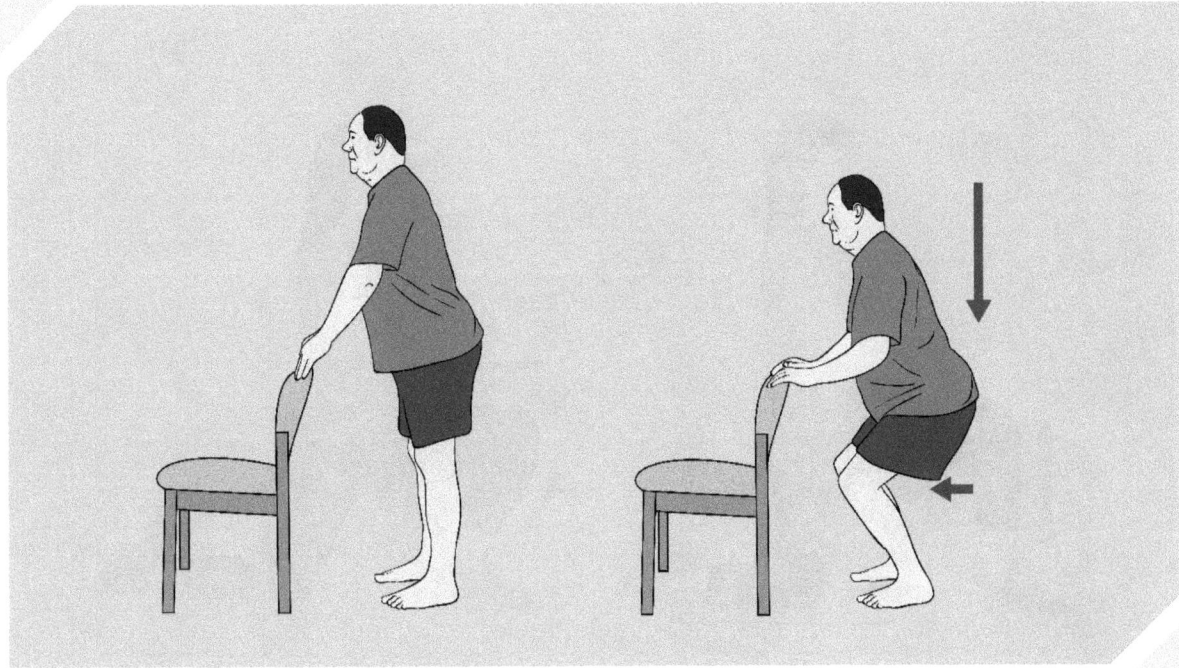

# INNER THIGH STRETCH

**Time Needed:** Two minutes

## Directions:

1. Stand up tall with your hands resting on a countertop or sturdy chair. Your feet should be apart as wide as comfortable with toes pointing outwards.

2. Bend at the knees as you bring your torso down into a squat with both knees pointing outwards. Only go as low as comfortable. Hold the stretch for 10 seconds. Rise back up to a standing position.

3. Repeat the stretch five more times.

**Cautions:** Only go as low into the position as is comfortable. Take care not to strain these inner muscles.

**Level Up:** To make this more challenging, hold the stretch for 20 or 30 seconds. You can also use just one hand, fingertips, or no hands for support.

**Benefits:** Improves flexibility and range of motion in the inner thigh and groin.

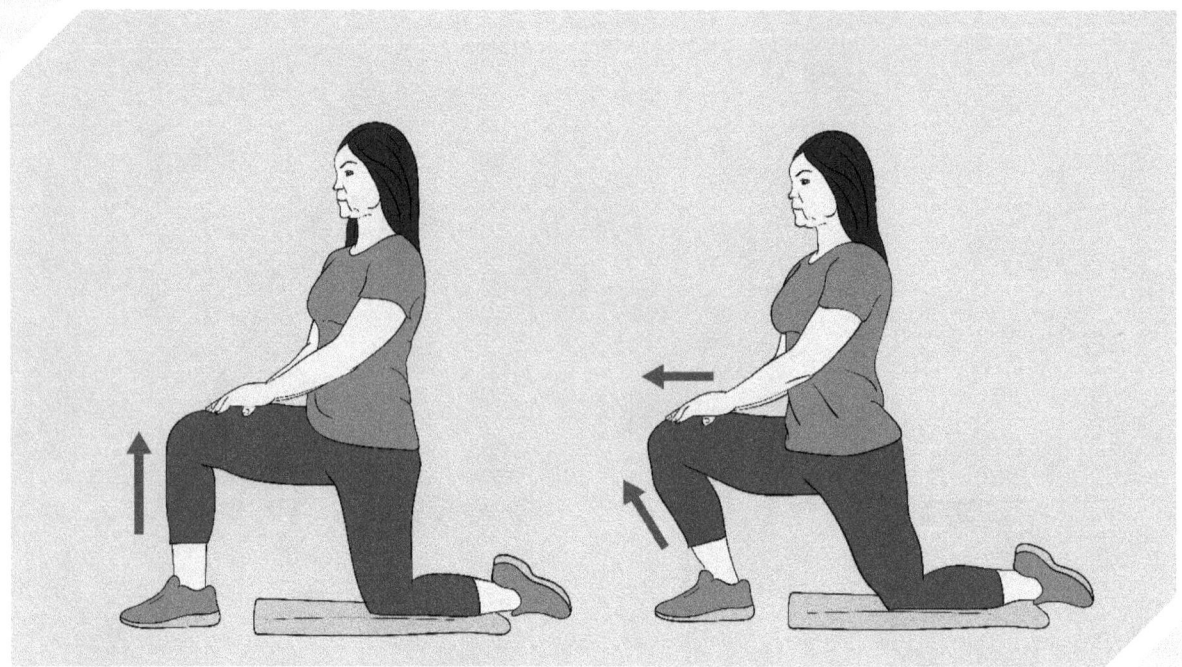

# KNEELING HIP FLEXOR STRETCH

## Time Needed: Four minutes

### Directions:

1. Kneel on a padded mat. The right knee should be on the mat and below the right hip. Bring the left knee up so that the left foot is on the floor and the left knee is directly above it. Both knees should be at 90-degree angles.

2. Tighten your core and move your body forward while bending your left knee further. Your spine should be straight and not bent forward. You should feel the stretch in the front part of your right hip. Hold for 30 seconds, then slowly return to the starting position. Repeat the stretch on this side two more times.

3. Change legs, now with the left knee on the mat and the right knee up. Complete the move a total of three times on the left side.

**Cautions:** Keep your pelvis straight and square as you lean into the forward bent knee to ensure the hip flexor gets stretched. You can put extra padding under the knee that is on the ground if needed.

**Level Up:** As you get stronger, you can increase the time spent in the stretch from 30 seconds to 45 seconds or one minute.

**Benefits:** Increases flexibility in the front of the hips.

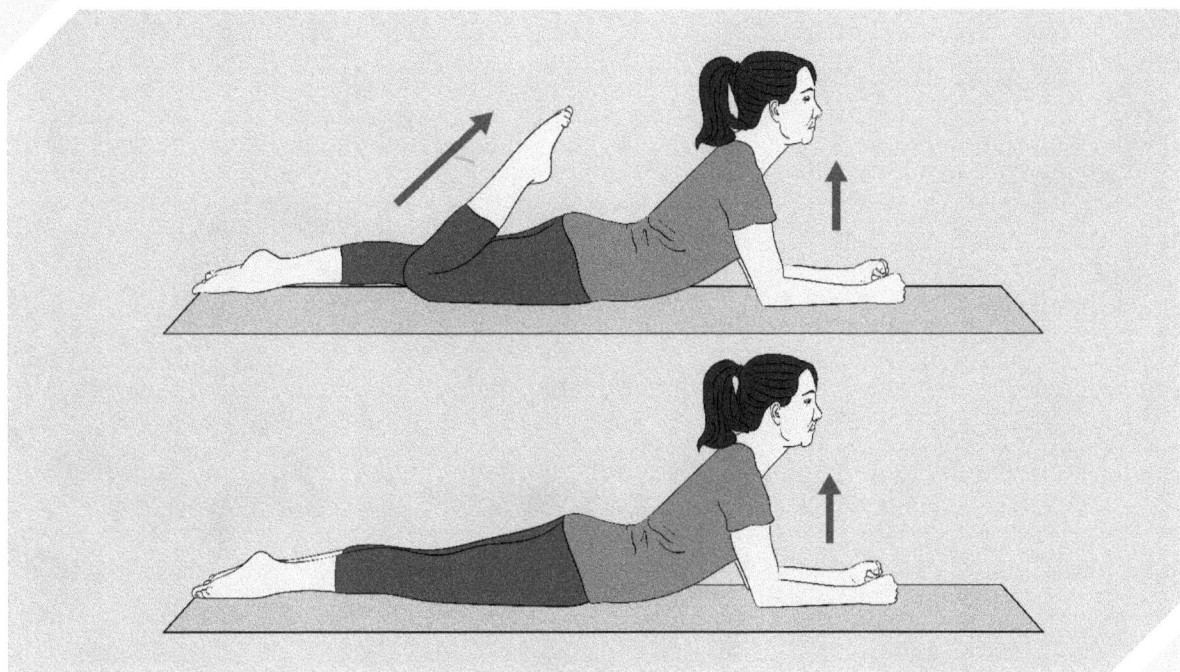

# ONE LEG KICK

**Time Needed:** One minute

## Directions:

1. Lie face down on a padded mat. Legs should be together and straight, toes pointed behind you. Raise your upper body up and support it with your forearms on the mat and elbows directly under your shoulders.

2. Bend your right knee and kick your right foot towards your right buttock twice. Return the right foot to the starting position.

3. Now, bend your left knee and kick your left foot towards your left buttock twice. Return the left foot to the starting position. This is one set.

4. Repeat for four more sets.

**Cautions:** Do not arch your lower back. Keep your spine long and pelvis pressed to the mat.

**Level Up:** Increase the number of sets to 10 or more.

**Benefits:** Helps back extensors and hamstrings strengthen and remain flexible.

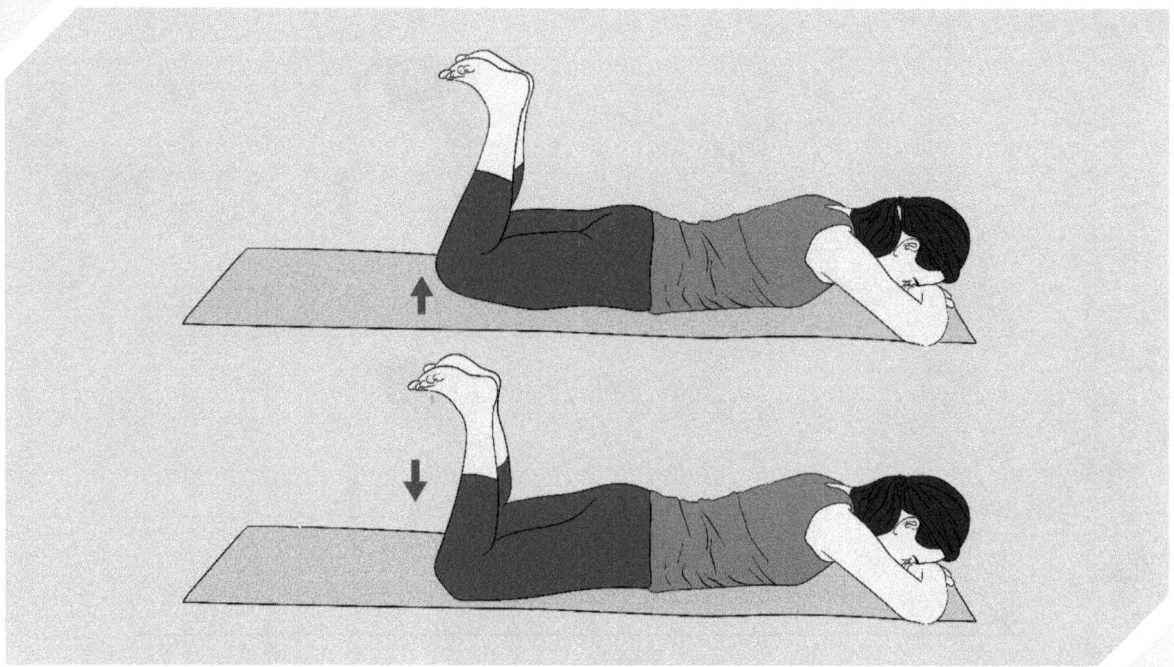

# PRONE HEEL SQUEEZE

## Time Needed: Two minutes

## Directions:

1. Lie face down on a padded mat. Place your palms down on the mat and allow your forehead to rest on top of them. Press your shoulders away from your ears.

2. Bend your knees so that the inner side of the knees are in contact with the floor and the outer knees are facing out to the sides. Flex both feet and bring your heels together in the air.

3. Draw your breath in and engage your core. As you exhale, squeeze your glutes. Inhale again and relax.

4. Repeat Step 3 for five more times.

**Cautions:** Do not touch your toes together, only your heels should touch. Don't hold your breath while performing this exercise.

**Level Up:** As you get stronger, increase the reps to 10 or more.

**Benefits:** Increases flexibility in the hips as well as toning your glutes.

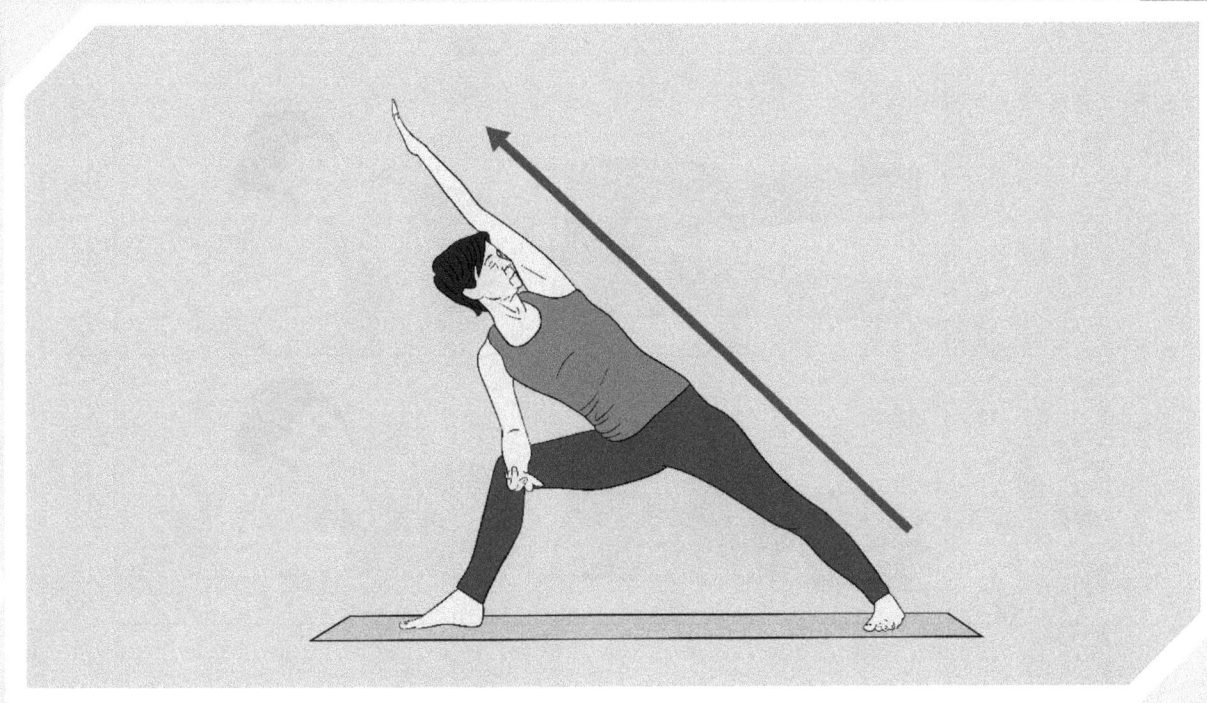

# SIDE ANGLE POSE

## Time Needed: Three minutes

### Directions:

1. Stand up tall with your legs wide and your toes pointing in front of you. Turn your right foot 90 degrees so that it points outward to the right.

2. Slowly bend your right knee as you bring your right forearm down to the top of your right thigh. Lift your left arm up over your head and stretch to the right so that your left upper arm is just above your left ear. Maintain this position for 20 seconds. Slowly rise back up to an upright position. Do this two more times.

3. Now, switch sides. Your left foot will turn out towards the left. Slowly bend your left knee and as you bring your left forearm on the top of your left thigh. Stretch your right arm up and over your head just above your right ear. Do this pose a total of three times.

**Cautions:** Keep your spine straight and lifted. Do not allow your back to round or flex forward.

**Level Up:** As you get stronger, hold the position for 30 seconds or longer.

**Benefits:** Helps to stretch the obliques and side body as well as legs.

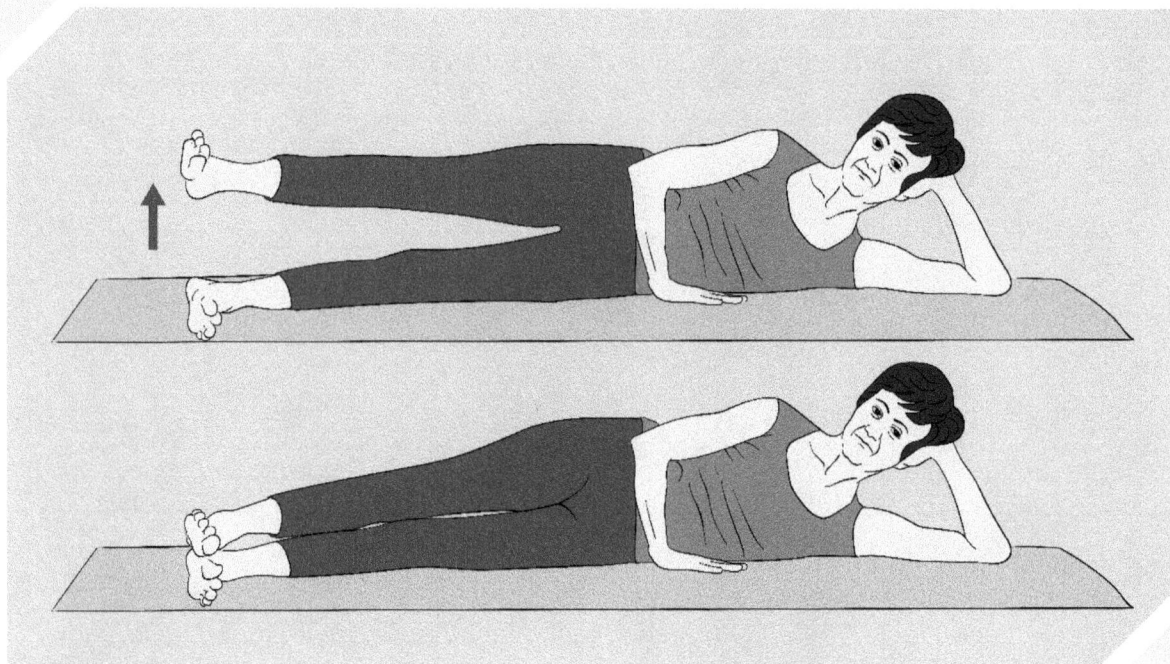

# SIDE KICK

**Time Needed:** Two minutes

## Directions:

1. Lie on a padded mat on your right side. Hips should be stacked one on top of the other. Shoulder, hips, and angles should form a straight line.

2. Either prop your head up with your right hand and right arm bent, or if this bothers your neck you can lay your head down on your right upper arm. The left hand is on the mat in front of you for support.

3. Kick your left leg forward and pulse twice before sweeping it to the back once. Immediately repeat the move four more times on this leg.

4. Switch sides by rolling onto your left side. Repeat the move on the left a total of five times.

**Cautions:** Do not allow your lower back to arch when you sweep your leg back behind you. Keep your spine long and straight.

**Level Up:** As you get stronger, increase the number of reps to 10 or more.

**Benefits:** Helps flexibility, strength, and mobility in your back extensors, hips, and glutes.

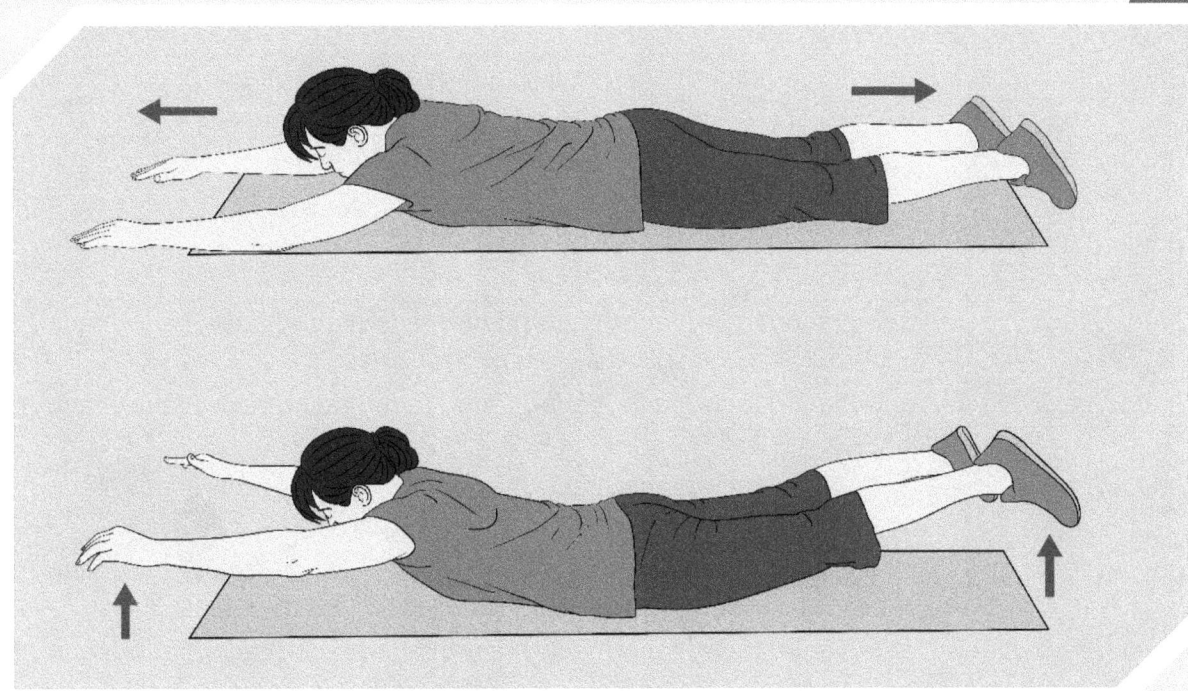

# SUPERMAN POSE

**Time Needed:** Three minutes

## Directions:

1. Lie down on a mat, face down. Extend your legs straight and arms straight overhead. Keep your shoulders down away from your ears.

2. Engage your core and glutes as you lift your hands a few inches off the mat. Bring them down, then lift your feet a few inches off the mat. Continue alternating lifting hands and then feet for a total of 10 times each.

**Cautions:** Keep your neck long and gaze down at the floor to avoid neck strain.

**Level Up:** Once you are comfortable with this move, make it more challenging by lifting your hands and feet off the mat at the same time.

**Benefits:** Strengthens core and back muscles and keeps them flexible.

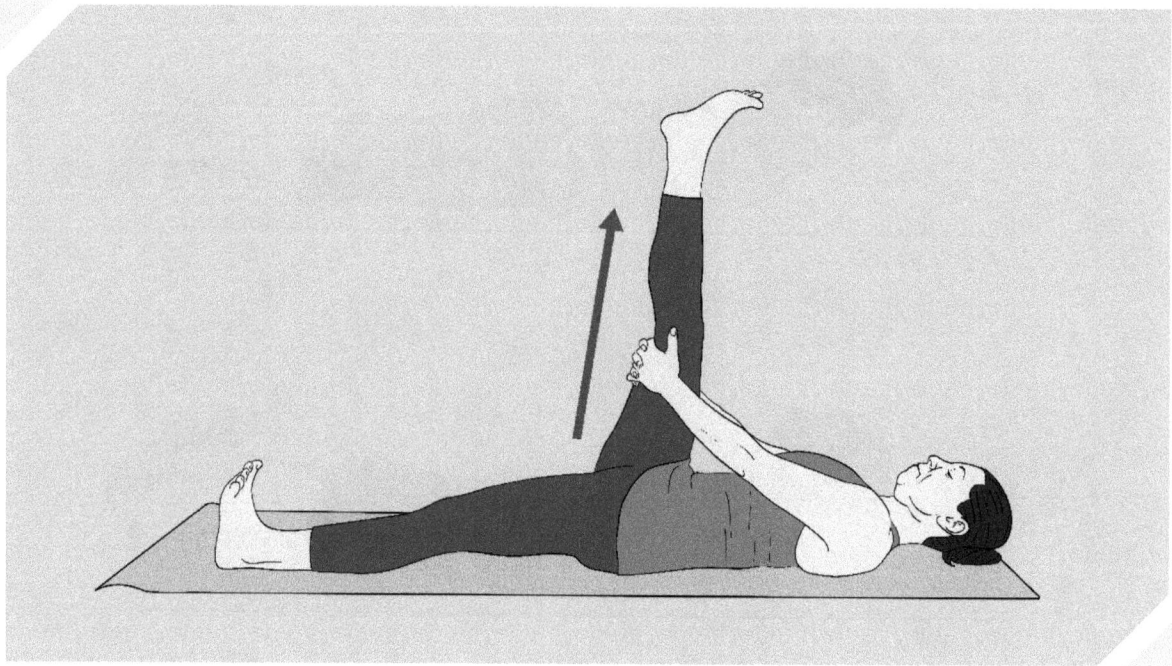

# SUPINE HAND-TO-BIG TOE

## Time Needed: Two minutes

### Directions:

1. Lie down on a mat with your face towards the ceiling. Keep legs straight and flex both feet.

2. Lift up your right leg up until it is vertical and perpendicular to the floor. Depending on your flexibility, try to bring your leg closer to your chest if you are able. You can use a strap or belt to assist you. Maintain the pose for five seconds, then slowly lower your leg back down to the floor.

3. Switch legs by lifting up your left leg up to the vertical position. Hold for five seconds then lower. This is one set.

4. Perform the movement for four more sets.

**Cautions:** Be extra careful to not allow your head and neck to lift off the floor or to crane forward. Allow the lower back to keep its natural lumbar curve by not pressing your lower back into the floor.

**Level Up:** Once your hamstrings are more flexible bring your leg closer to your chest while keeping your pelvis straight and square.

**Benefits:** Stretches the hamstrings and lower back.

# Chapter 3:
# Improving Your Posture

Take a quick glance at yourself in the mirror or window. Are your shoulders slumped forward and your upper back rounded? Inhale and straighten up as you roll your shoulders back. Notice a difference? You look taller and appear more confident. But you also have protected your back and spine while improving blood flow by doing this.

> Number one, like yourself. Number two, you have to eat healthy. And number three, you've got to squeeze your buns. That's my formula.
>
> **Richard Simmons**

Proper posture is important for people of any age, but especially for those over 50 years old. Good posture increases circulation, strengthens back muscles, and lifts your spirits. Many exercises to improve posture involve strengthening your core. The muscles in your torso are responsible for helping your body maintain good posture so it is important to keep those exercised and strong. These same exercises also help alleviate and prevent lower back pain that is due to poor posture.

In this chapter, we will perform twelve exercises to build and maintain a good posture position. No equipment is needed, but access to a mat and sturdy chair or wall is helpful.

# POSTURE EXERCISES

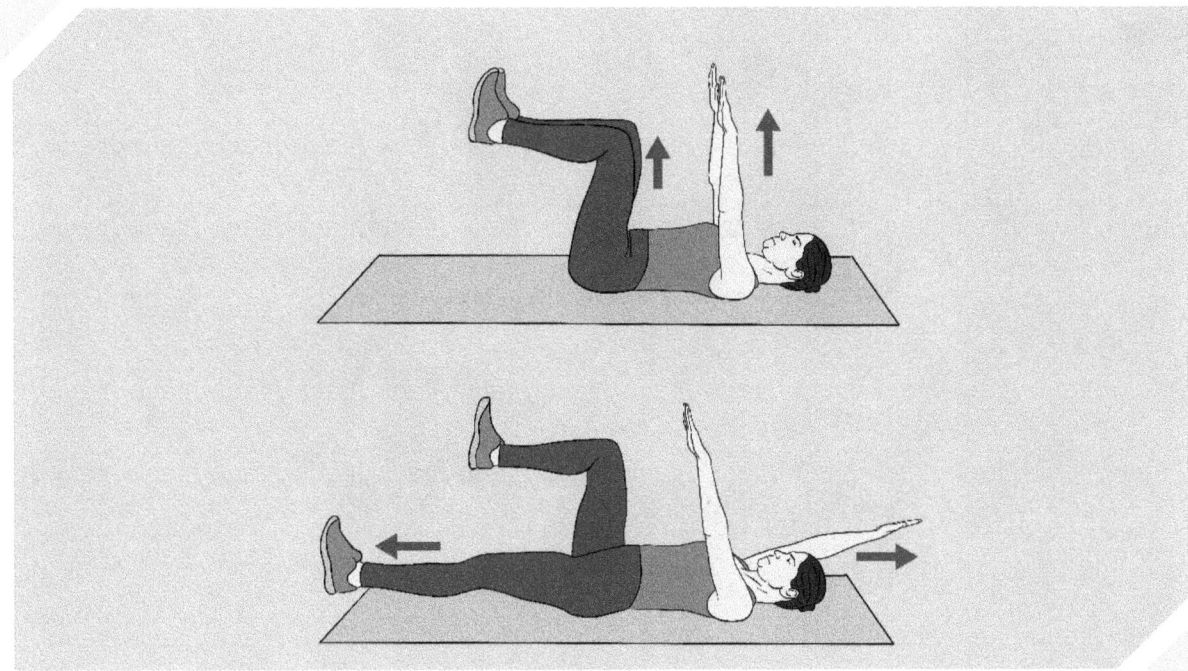

# DEAD BUG

**Time Needed:** Three minutes

## Directions:

1.  Lie down on a mat on your back. Bend your knees and raise them so they are directly above your hips. Lift your feet so that shins are parallel to the floor and knees are at a 90-degree angle.

2.  Bring arms straight up towards the ceiling. Tighten your core muscles as you straighten your left leg down to the floor and your right arm over your head. Slowly bring your arm and leg back to the starting position.

3.  Repeat the same motion with your right leg and left arm. This is one set.

4.  Repeat the exercise on alternating sides for four more sets.

**Cautions:** Keep your lower back pressed into the floor and your core engaged as you perform the exercise.

**Level Up:** To make this more challenging as you get stronger, don't let your arms and legs touch the floor when they are straight. Keep them hovering just above the floor.

**Benefits:** Strengthens your core muscles and helps posture.

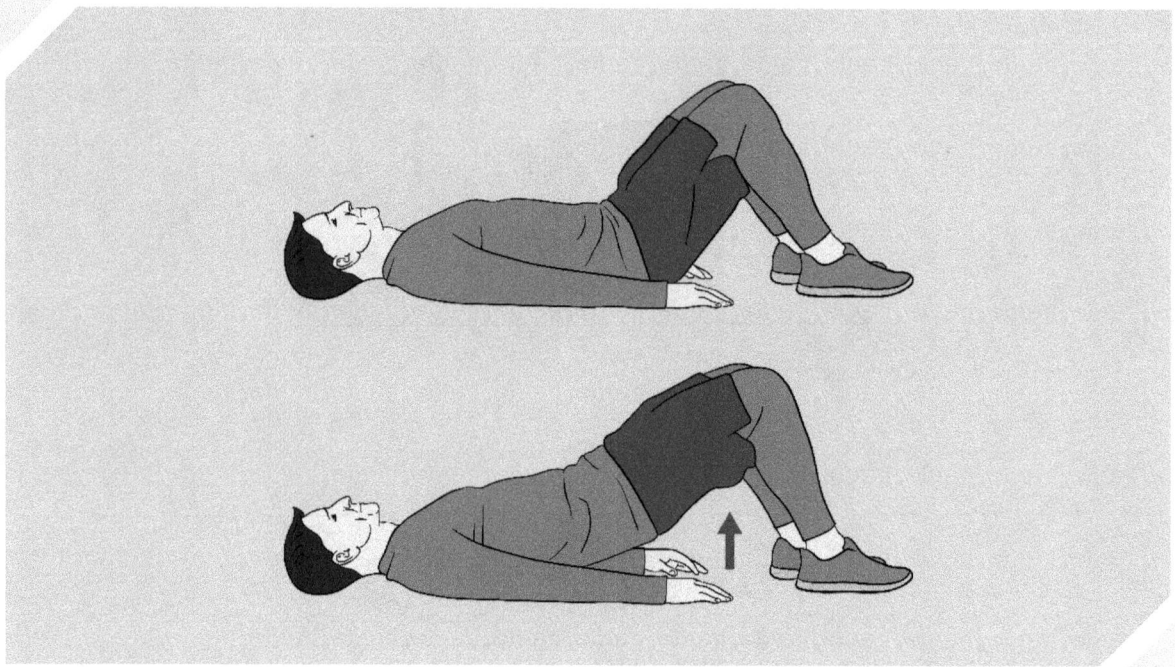

# GLUTE BRIDGE

**Time Needed:** Two minutes

## Directions:

1. Lie down on a mat with your face towards the ceiling. Bend your knees and keep your feet flat on the floor. Legs should be hip-width apart and arms down by your sides on the floor.

2. Tighten your core and glutes as you lift your hips straight up towards the ceiling. Shoulders, hips, and knees should form a straight diagonal line that looks like a bridge. Pause, then slowly lower to the starting position.

3. Repeat the move for a total of 10 times.

**Cautions:** Keep your neck long and your head on the ground while performing this move. Don't hunch up your shoulders but keep them pressed down.

**Level Up:** You can make this harder by lifting one foot off the floor while in the bridge position.

**Benefits:** Works to tighten and strengthen your core, glutes, hamstrings, and lower back.

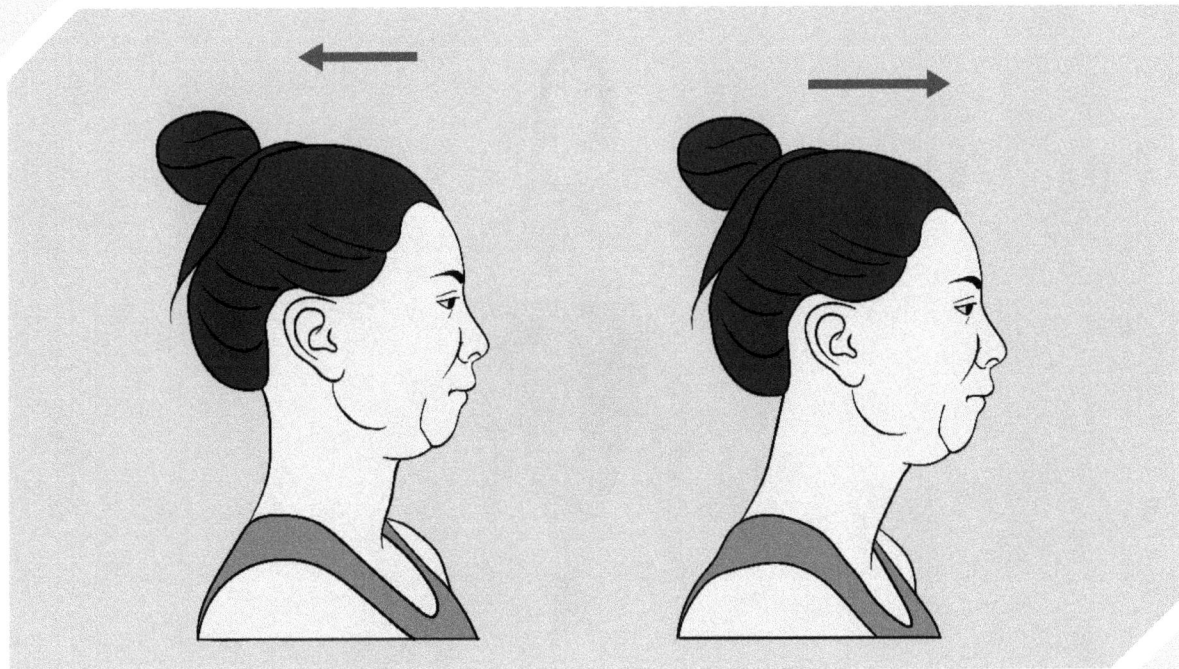

# HEAD PRESS

**Time Needed:** Two minutes

## Directions:

1. Sit up straight with your arms relaxed and down by your side and feet flat on the floor.

2. Press your head back as far as possible without tilting your chin down. Hold for two seconds then return to the starting position.

3. Repeat the move a total of 10 times.

**Cautions:** Do not lean back while pressing your head back. Hold onto a chair or counter if you need help with balance.

**Level Up:** Do this exercise standing with your back against a wall. Press your head back against the wall.

**Benefits:** Helps to loosen neck muscles and align your head and shoulders.

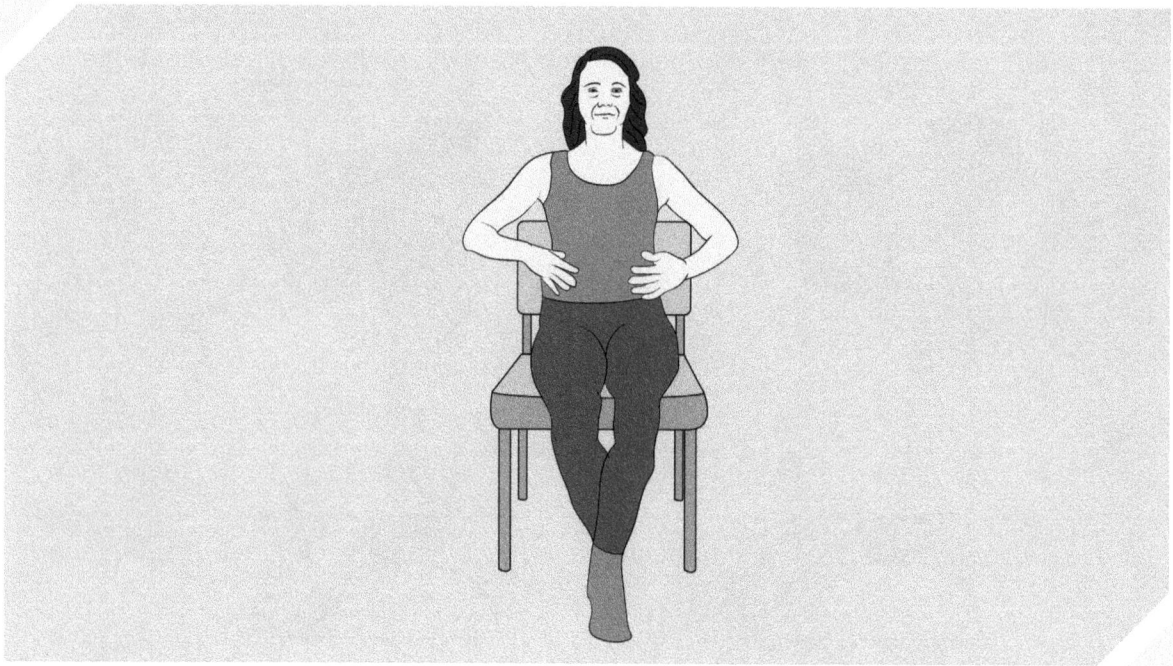

# ISOMETRIC ABDOMINALS

**Time Needed:** One minute

## Directions:

1. Sit up tall in a sturdy chair with back support. Your feet should be flat on the floor and your arms down by your sides.

2. Engage the muscles in your core and tighten them. Bring both hands to your abdominals and press your fingers as you tighten your core muscles further. Hold for 10 seconds. Rest then repeat four more times.

**Cautions:** Don't hold your breath when tightening core muscles and do not lean forward.

**Level Up:** To make this more challenging, do this move while standing.

**Benefits:** Strengthens core muscles and torso support for good posture.

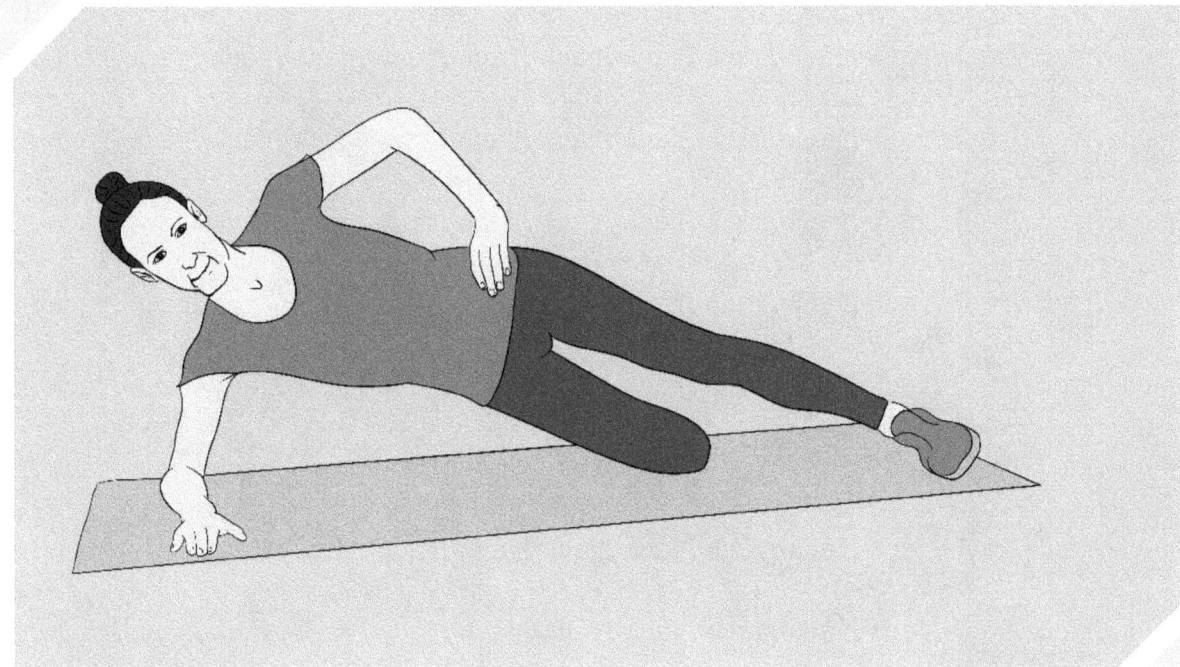

# MODIFIED FOREARM SIDE PLANK

## Time Needed: Two minutes

## Directions:

1. Lie on a mat on your right side with hips stacked one above the other. Shoulders, hips, and ankles should be in a straight line.

2. Bend your right arm and bring your elbow so it is under your right shoulder. Bend your right knee at a 90-degree angle so that your right foot is behind you.

3. Engage your core muscles as you lift your body up onto your right forearm and right knee, keeping your body in a straight line. Return slowly to the starting position. Repeat on this side three times in total.

4. Switch sides and repeat the exercise on the left side three times.

**Cautions:** Do not allow your hips to sag or lift high.

**Level Up:** Once you are comfortable doing this, try doing it with both legs straight when you lift your body.

**Benefits:** Strengthens your entire core to help maintain good posture.

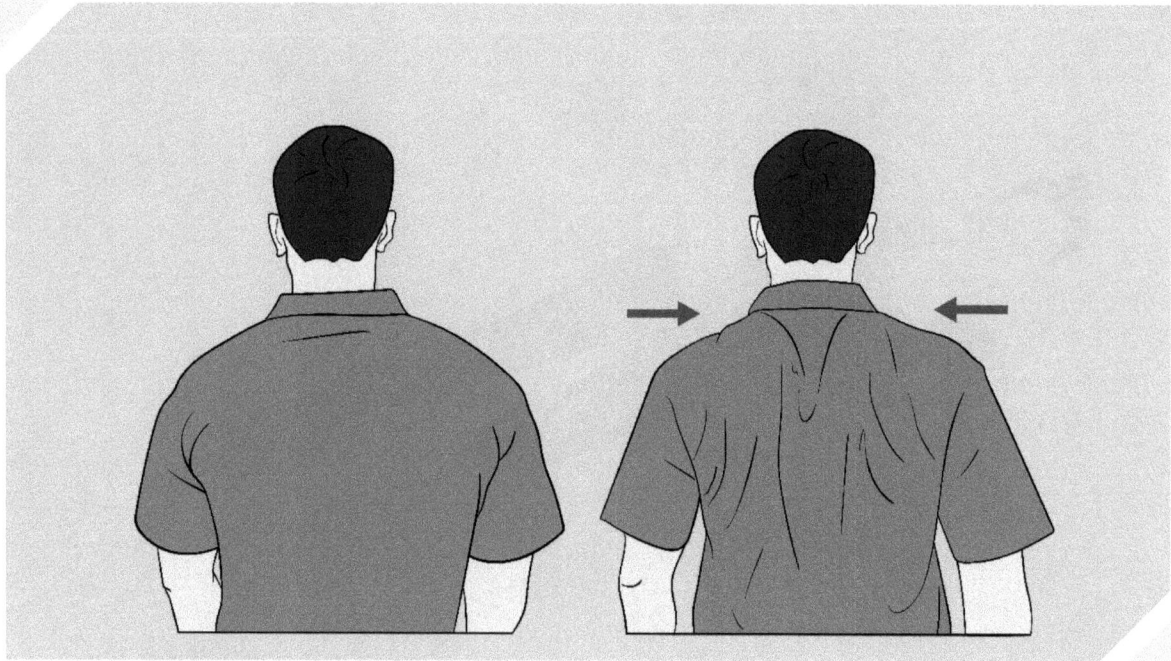

# SHOULDER BLADE SQUEEZE

## Time Needed: One minute

### Directions:

1. Place your buttocks onto the seat of a sturdy chair while keeping your feet flat on the floor. Bend your elbows.

2. Squeeze your shoulder blades together as you move both elbows towards the back of the chair and behind you. Pause, then return arms back to the original position.

3. Repeat the move for a total of 10 times.

**Cautions:** Do not lift your shoulders while performing this move. Keep them down and away from your ears.

**Level Up:** Do this exercise standing and increase the number of reps.

**Benefits:** This works the central muscles of the back that surround the spine.

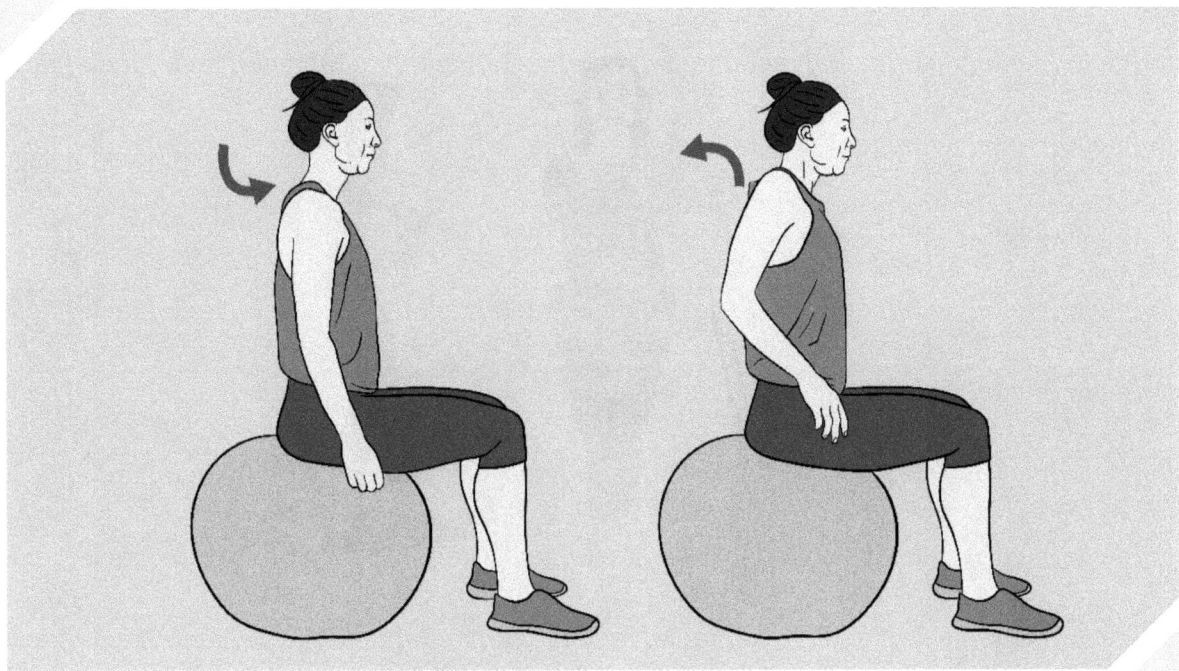

# SHOULDER ROLLS

**Time Needed:** One minute

## Directions:

1. Sit up tall in a chair with your arms relaxed and down by your side. The feet are flat on the floor.

2. Raise your shoulders up towards your ears then backward and down to their starting position in one smooth circular motion. Repeat for a total of 10 times.

**Cautions:** Don't clench your jaw while performing shoulder rolls. Keep your jaw and face relaxed.

**Level Up:** Do this exercise standing with feet hip-width apart.

**Benefits:** Helps to loosen shoulders and upper back and counter any forward hunching.

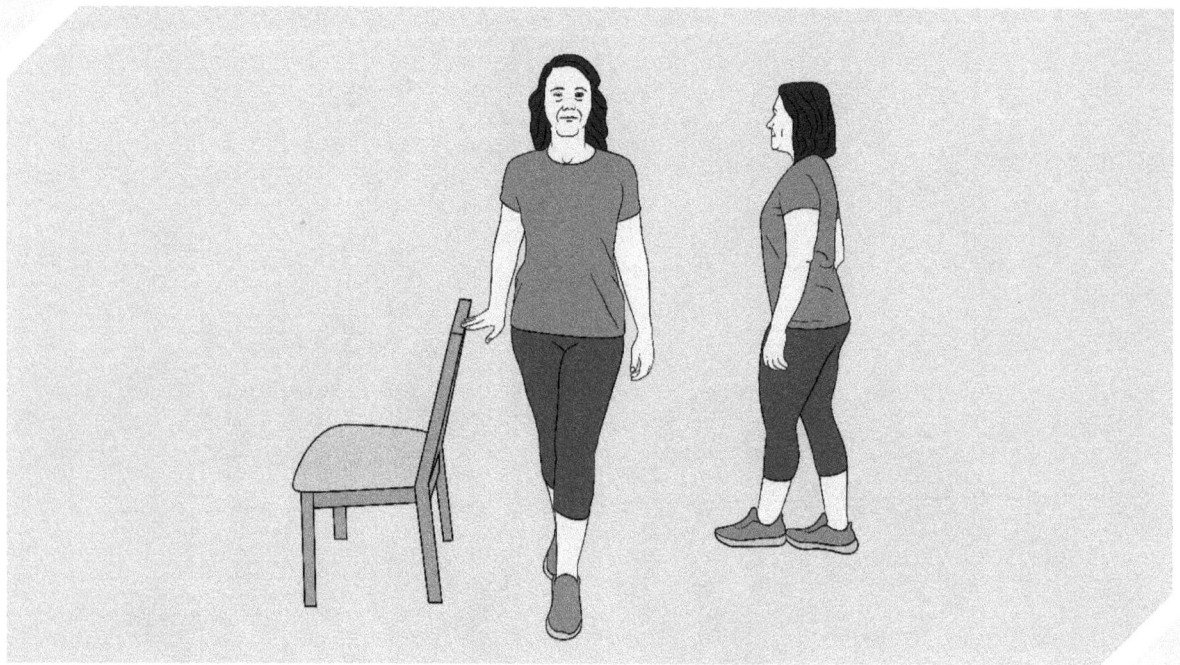

# TANDEM STAND

## Time Needed: Two minutes

## Directions:

1. Stand sideways next to a wall, countertop, or sturdy chair with one hand on the stable object for support.

2. Place your right foot directly in front of your left one with your right heel and left toes touching, as if you were walking on a tightrope. Hold the position for 10 seconds. Return to the starting position, then repeat for a total of five times.

3. Switch sides by now placing the left foot in front of the right and holding the position. Do the move five times on the left.

**Cautions:** Keep your spine erect and core engaged. Don't lean too far on either leg.

**Level Up:** To make this more difficult, try it with your eyes closed. You can also not hold onto the wall for support.

**Benefits:** Helps to improve posture as well as balance.

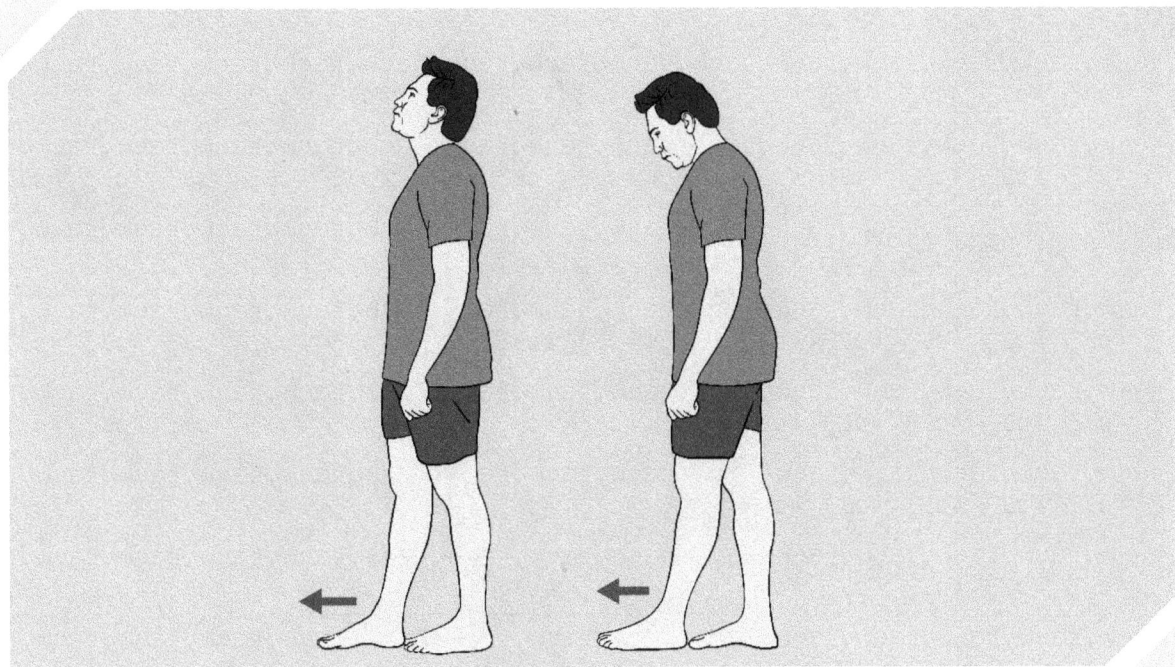

# TANDEM WALK

## Time Needed: Two minutes

### Directions:

1. Stand sideways next to a wall or long countertop. Place one hand on it for support.

2. Put your right foot directly in front of your left with the right heel touching the left toes.

3. Walk forward, doing the same thing with your left foot in front. Continue walking for 10 steps. Turn around and walk back. This is one set.

4. Repeat for two more sets.

**Cautions:** Be aware of any tripping hazards and move them out of your path before starting.

**Level Up:** Make this more difficult by not holding on with your hand for support.

**Benefits:** Helps to improve posture and balance.

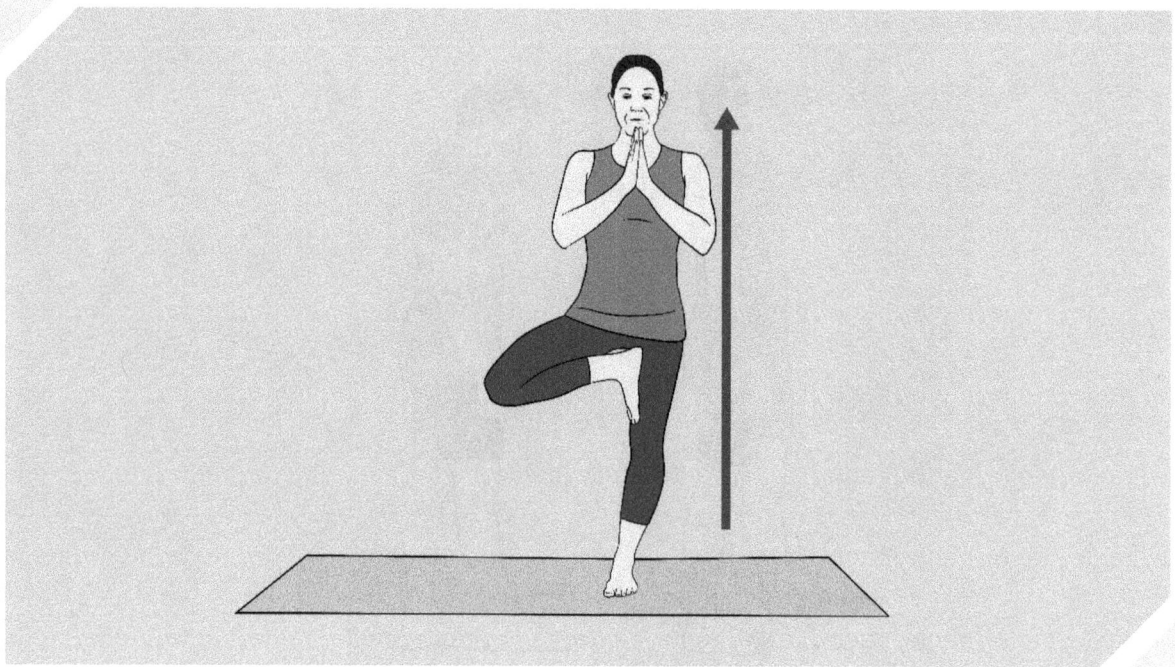

# TREE POSE

## Time Needed: Three minutes

### Directions:

1. Stand up straight next to a wall, countertop, or sturdy chair and place one hand on it for support. Keep your feet directly below your hip bones.

2. Simultaneously lift your left foot and bend at your left knee. Now, bring the sole of your foot and place it on the inside of your right shin or right thigh, whichever is more comfortable for you. Pause, then lower the foot back down to the ground. Repeat four more times.

3. Switch legs. Bend your right knee and place your right foot on your left shin or thigh. Do this move five times.

**Cautions:** Avoid placing your foot on the inside of your knee, especially if you have any knee issues.

**Level Up:** This is more challenging if you do not hold onto anything for support. Hands can be at your hips, out to the sides, or above your head. Keep your eyes fixed on an unmoving object in front of you to help with balance.

**Benefits:** Aids in balance and good posture.

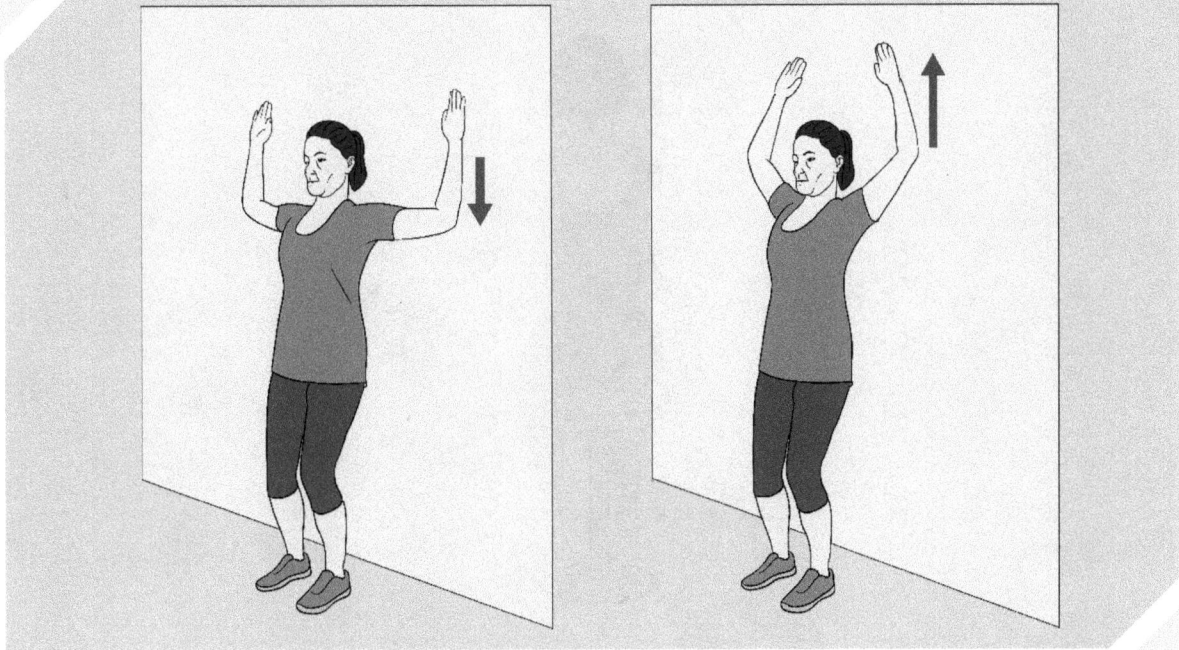

# WALL ANGELS

**Time Needed:** One minute

## Directions:

1. Stand up straight with your back against a wall. Shoulders, glutes, and heels should be in contact with the wall. Knees can be slightly bent.

2. Lift both arms and bend at the elbows 90 degrees into a cactus shape with the backs of your hands touching the wall.

3. Straighten both arms as you slide your hands up the wall above your head. Slowly bring them back down to starting position. Repeat a total of five times.

**Cautions:** Keep your head and neck in a neutral position and not craned forward.

**Level Up:** As you get used to the exercise increase the repetitions to 10 or more.

**Benefits:** Opens the chest and increases flexibility in the shoulders and upper back to help maintain good posture.

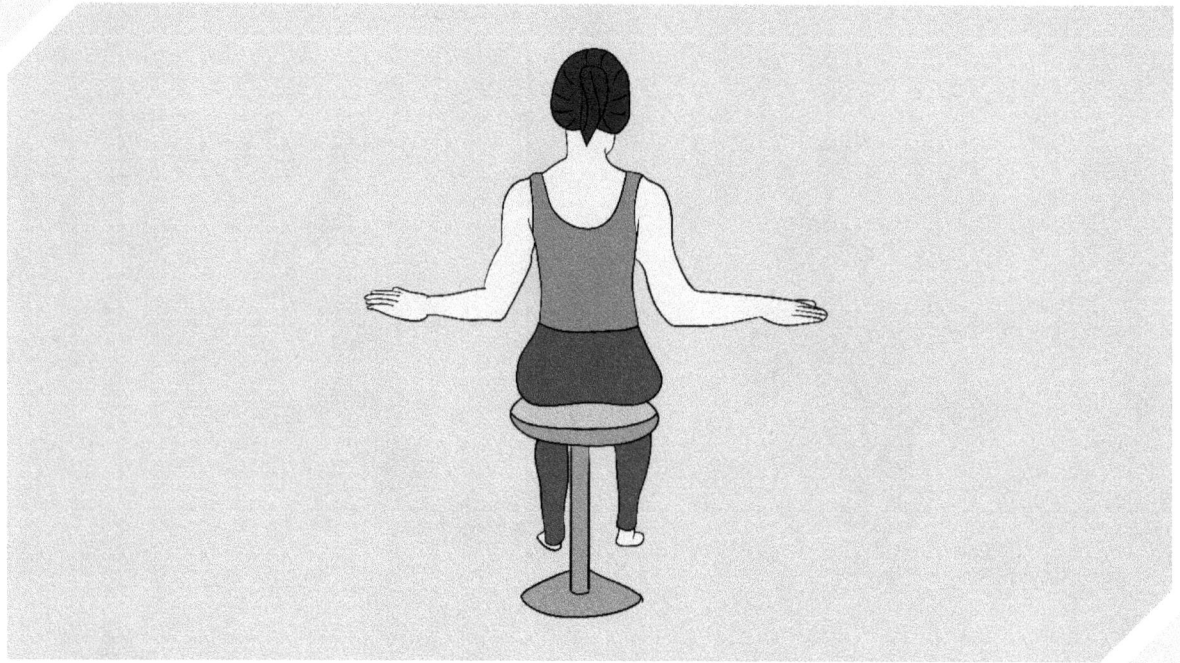

# WAXING

**Time Needed:** Two minutes

## Directions:

1. Sit up tall in a sturdy chair with back support. Your feet should be flat on the floor and your arms down by your sides.

2. Bend both elbows so they form a 90-degree angle. Press the upper arms and elbows into your sides with your palms facing down toward the floor.

3. Squeeze your shoulder blades together as you move your hands and forearms in a semi-circular motion as if you were applying wax to a car or furniture. Keep waxing for 30 seconds. Rest then repeat four more times.

**Cautions:** Don't hunch up your neck and shoulders. Keep your shoulders pressed down and away from your ears.

**Level Up:** For an extra challenge, do this exercise while standing.

**Benefits:** Strengthens your core and upper back to help with posture and alignment.

# Chapter 4:
# Improving Your Strength

Are you thinking that strength training involves lifting heavy weights? It can, but strengthening your muscles can be done with your own body weight or light hand weights just as effectively.

The mass of our larger muscles decreases with age. As we get older, it is important to replace lost muscle and build new muscle to maintain

> If you think lifting weights is dangerous, try being weak. Being weak is dangerous.
>
> **Bret Contreras**

our ability to do everyday tasks. Things like gardening, lifting groceries, playing with grandkids, and shopping all require a certain amount of strength and stamina.

Strength exercises are essential for maintaining and increasing muscle strength, especially the ones that support your spine. Many of these exercises are weight-bearing, meaning that they put good stress on your bones to help with bone density. Remember bones become more porous and weak if weight-bearing exercises are not done.

In this chapter, we will build strength with twelve exercises that challenge your muscles in a variety of ways. Some equipment is needed for these; including a mat, a sturdy chair, and two water bottles or light hand weights. Optional but not necessary equipment includes a pillow and resistance band

# STRENGTH EXERCISES

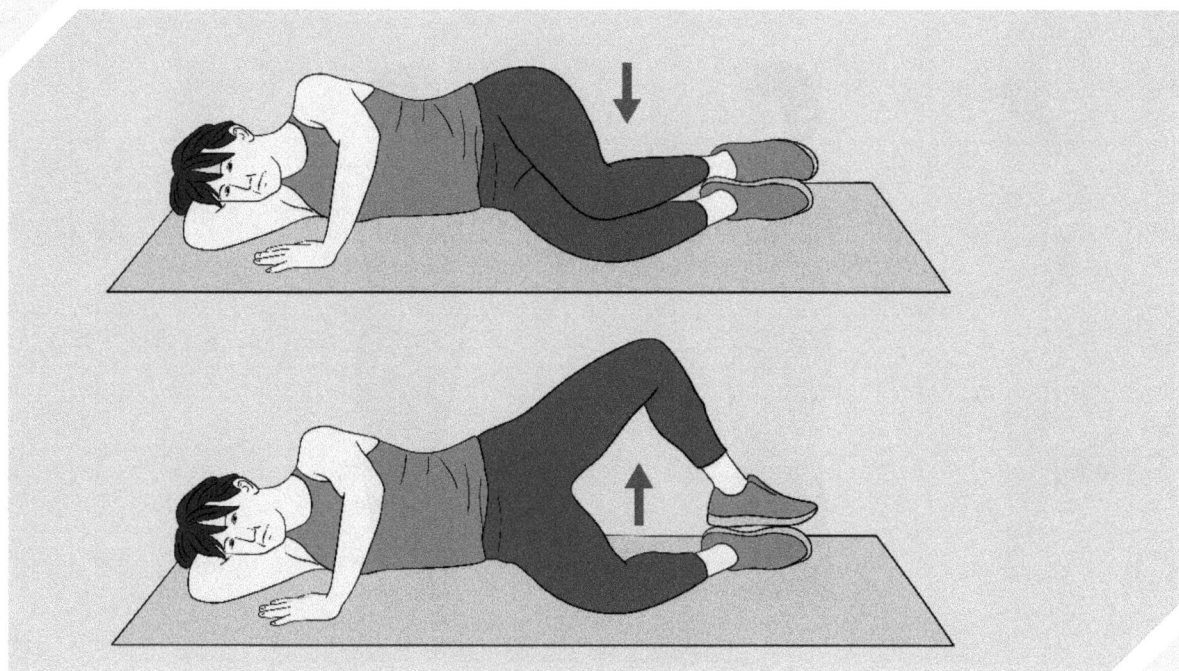

# CLAMSHELL

**Time Needed:** Two minutes

## Directions:

1. Lie on your right side on a padded mat. You can use a pillow to support your head if desired.

2. Bend both knees and keep feet together. Lift your right knee up and raise it toward the ceiling. Your upper body should not move and your lower leg and both feet should still be on the ground. Lower the knee back down to starting position. Repeat the move on this leg for a total of 10 times.

3. Switch sides by lying on your left side. Lift your left knee up toward the ceiling, keeping both feet together and on the mat. Repeat for 10 reps. This is one set.

4. Repeat to do two sets total.

**Cautions:** Do not rotate your spine or twist your upper body while doing this exercise.

**Level Up:** Once you are familiar with the exercise, add a small hand weight to the top leg to increase the resistance, or use a resistance band.

**Benefits:** Strengthens hips and the muscles surrounding the pelvis.

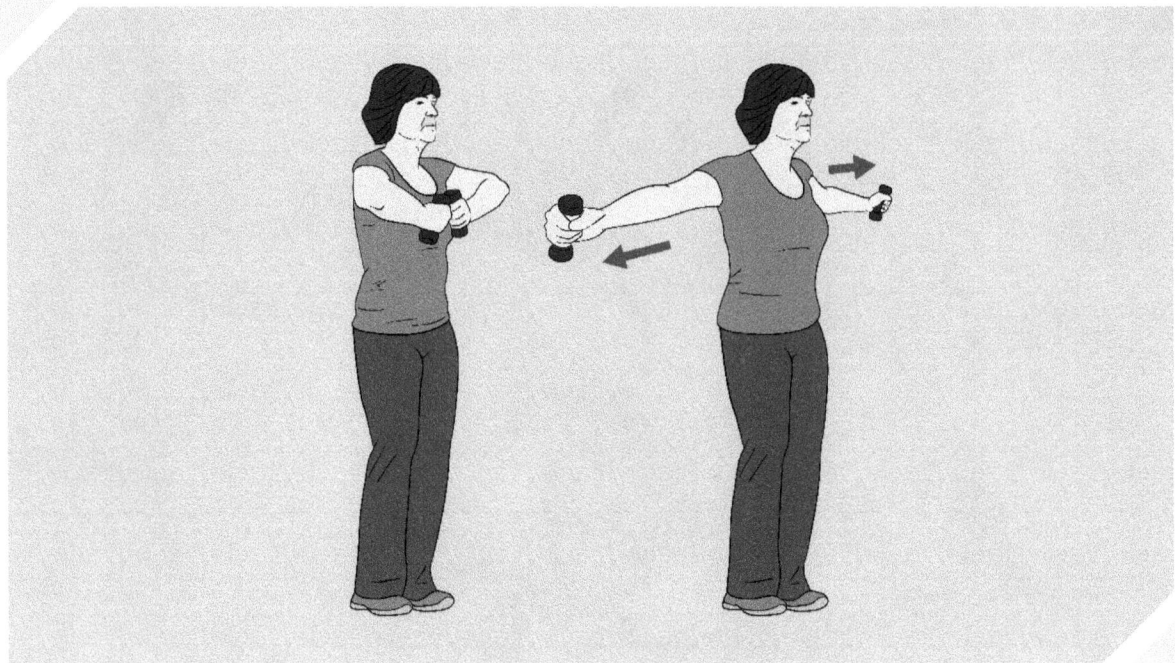

# ELBOW SIDE EXTENSIONS

## Time Needed: Two minutes

### Directions:

1. Stand up tall with your feet a hip-width distance apart. Hold water bottles or light hand weights in both hands.

2. Bend the elbows out to the sides as you bring the weights up to your chest with your palms facing toward you.

3. Straighten your right arm straight out to the right side so that it is perpendicular to the floor. Hold for 10 seconds and return your hand back to your chest. Repeat on this arm five more times.

4. Switch arms. Now straighten your left arm out to the left side and hold for 10 seconds before returning it to the starting position. Repeat on this arm five more times.

**Cautions:** Keep your spine straight and posture upright. Do not lean to either side while performing the exercise.

**Level Up:** As you get stronger, try straightening both arms out to the side at the same time. You can also increase the amount of weight.

**Benefits:** Strengthens your shoulders and upper arms while also improving your grip strength.

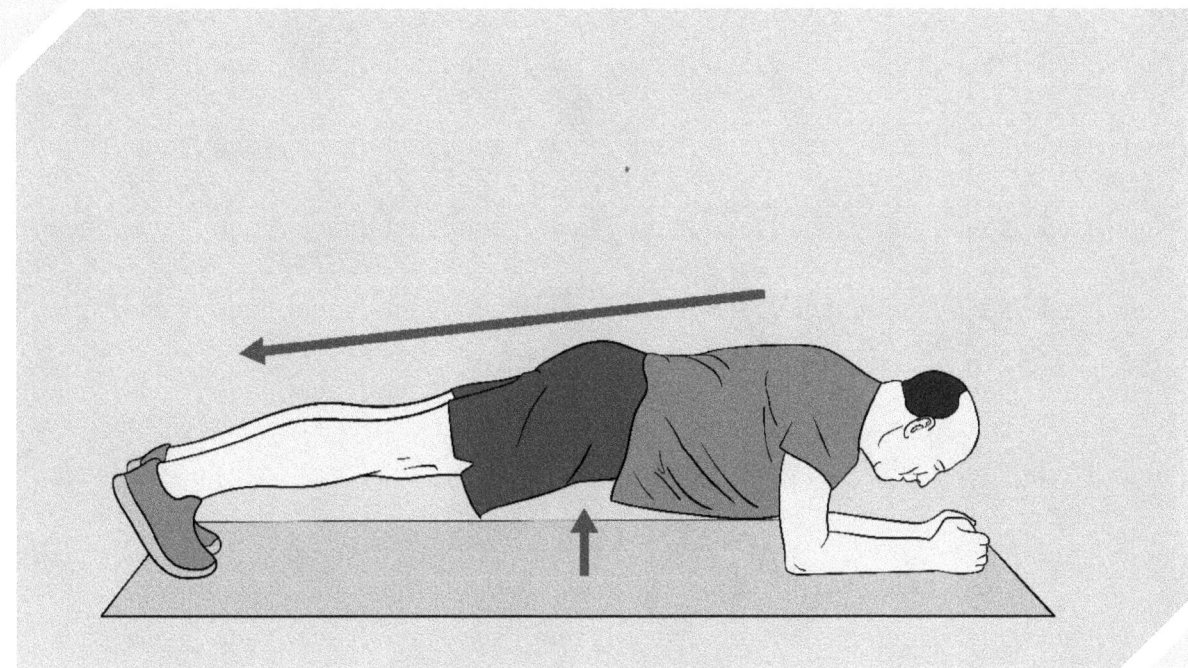

# FOREARM PLANK

## Time Needed: Two minutes

## Directions:

1. Get down on a mat on all fours. Place your forearms down on the mat with your elbows directly under your shoulders and hands in front of you.

2. Extend your legs, one by one, straight behind you so that you are supported by your toes. Keep your torso firm and lifted off the floor. Hold for a few seconds or as long as comfortable. Return to the starting position.

3. Repeat the plank five times.

**Cautions:** Don't hunch up your shoulders, keep them away from your ears. Be aware of your lower back and don't allow it to sag while in the plank position.

**Level Up:** For an extra challenge, hold the plank for longer periods of time. Work up to holding a plank for one minute, two minutes, or more.

**Benefits:** Works the core and shoulder muscles to strengthen them.

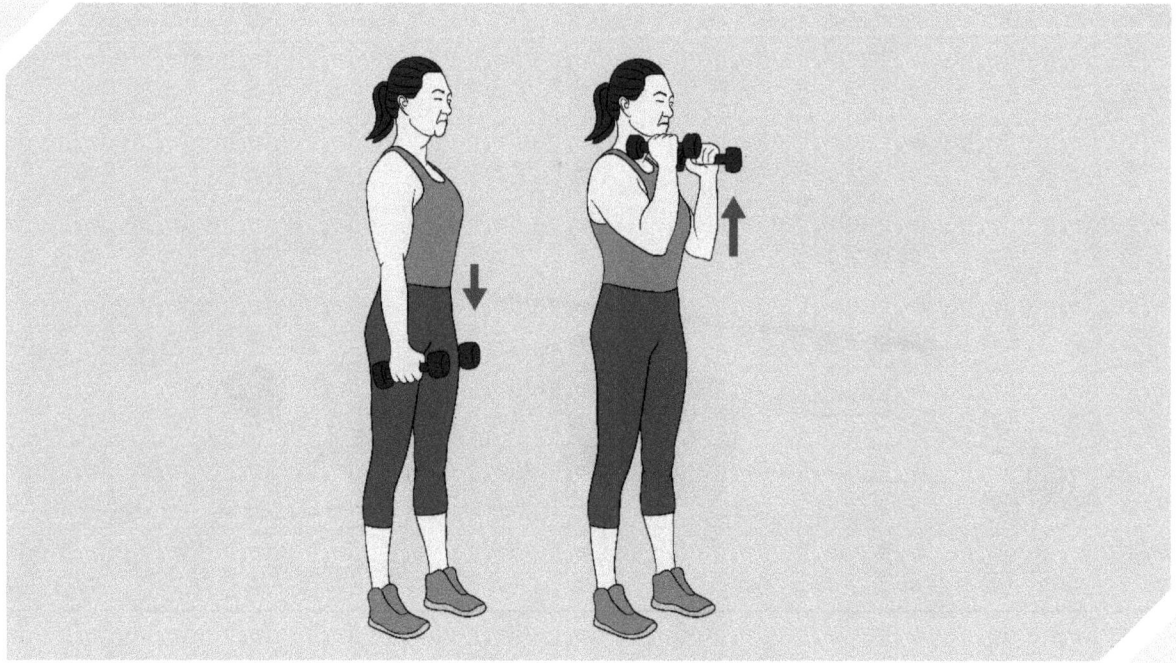

# HAMMER CURLS

**Time Needed:** Two minutes

## Directions:

1. Stand up tall with your feet directly below your hip bones. Grab two water bottles or hand weights in each hand. Place your hands down with your palms facing your thighs.

2. Keep your palms facing toward your thighs. Bring the weight up as far as you can towards your shoulder while you bend your right arm at the elbow. Try to keep the elbow close to the side of your body. Squeeze your right bicep as you do this. Lower your right hand back down to the starting position facing your thighs. Do a total of 10 reps.

3. Switch arms and bend your left elbow while lifting the weight towards your shoulder. Repeat for 10 reps.

**Cautions:** Be sure to keep your wrists aligned with your forearms and not bent inwards or outwards. Don't swing your arm but rather move in a slow and controlled movement.

**Level Up:** As you get stronger, you can increase the weight you are using or do both arms at the same time. You can also increase the number of reps.

**Benefits:** This variation of a bicep curl works more muscles in your arm than a traditional curl. It also targets wrists and grip strength.

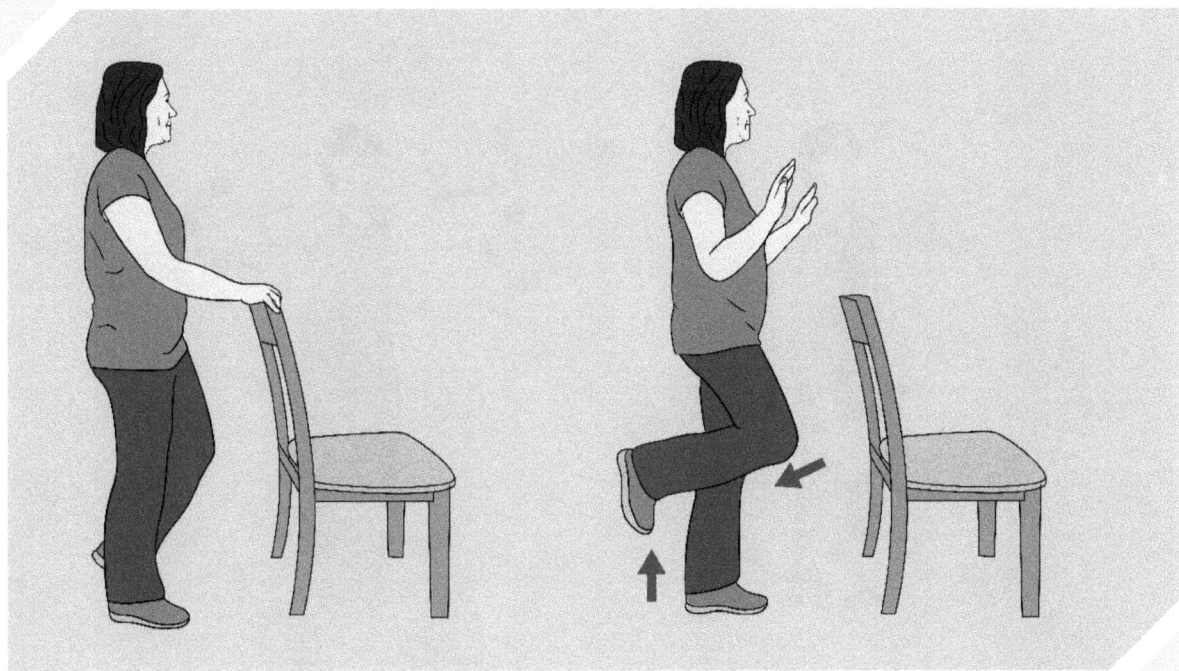

# HAMSTRING CURLS

**Time Needed:** Two minutes

## Directions:

1. Stand up straight next to a countertop or sturdy chair. Place both hands on it for support. Feet should be a hip-width distance apart.

2. Bend your right knee and lift your right foot behind you, keeping your thighs parallel. Flex your right foot and squeeze your right hamstring muscle. Slowly lower back to the starting position. Repeat this leg for a total of 10 times.

3. Switch legs. Bend your left knee and lift your left foot behind you while flexing your foot and squeezing the hamstring. Lower back to the starting position and repeat a total of 10 times. This is one set.

4. Repeat for a total of two sets.

**Cautions:** Do not swing the leg or use momentum to do the reps. Movements should be steady and controlled.

**Level Up:** Once you are stronger, you can increase the number of sets or add ankle weights to add resistance.

**Benefits:** This exercise helps to strengthen hamstrings and quads.

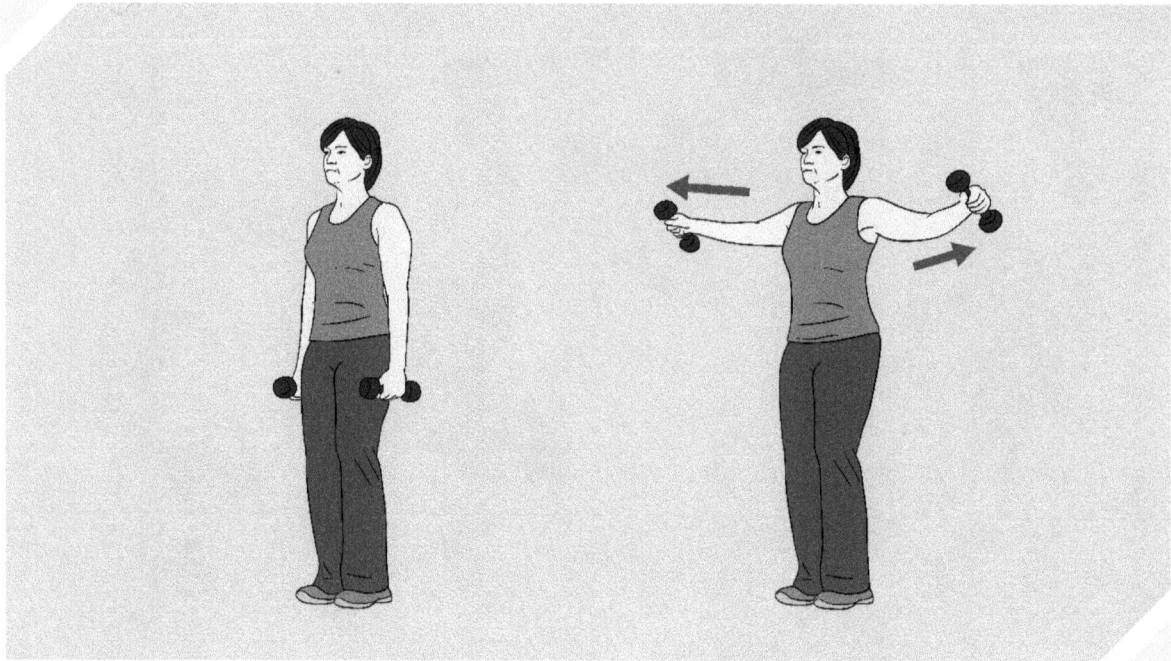

# LATERAL SHOULDER RAISE

## Time Needed: Two minutes

## Directions:

1. Stand with feet directly below your hip bones. Grab two water bottles or weights, one in each hand, and keep your arms down with your palms facing your thighs.

2. Engage your core as you lift your right arm out to the side away from your body. Lift your arm so that your hand is equal to shoulder height. Slowly lower your arm back down to its original position. Do this move a total of 10 times on this arm.

3. Switch arms. Raise your left arm out to the side with your left hand coming to shoulder height. Slowly lower your arm back down to its original position and repeat a total of 10 times. This is one set.

4. Repeat for three sets.

**Cautions:** Do not lean to one side or the other. Maintain an upright posture with your core tight.

**Level Up:** To make this more challenging, lift both arms at the same time.

**Benefits:** Strengthens the entire shoulder region and works the three deltoid muscles.

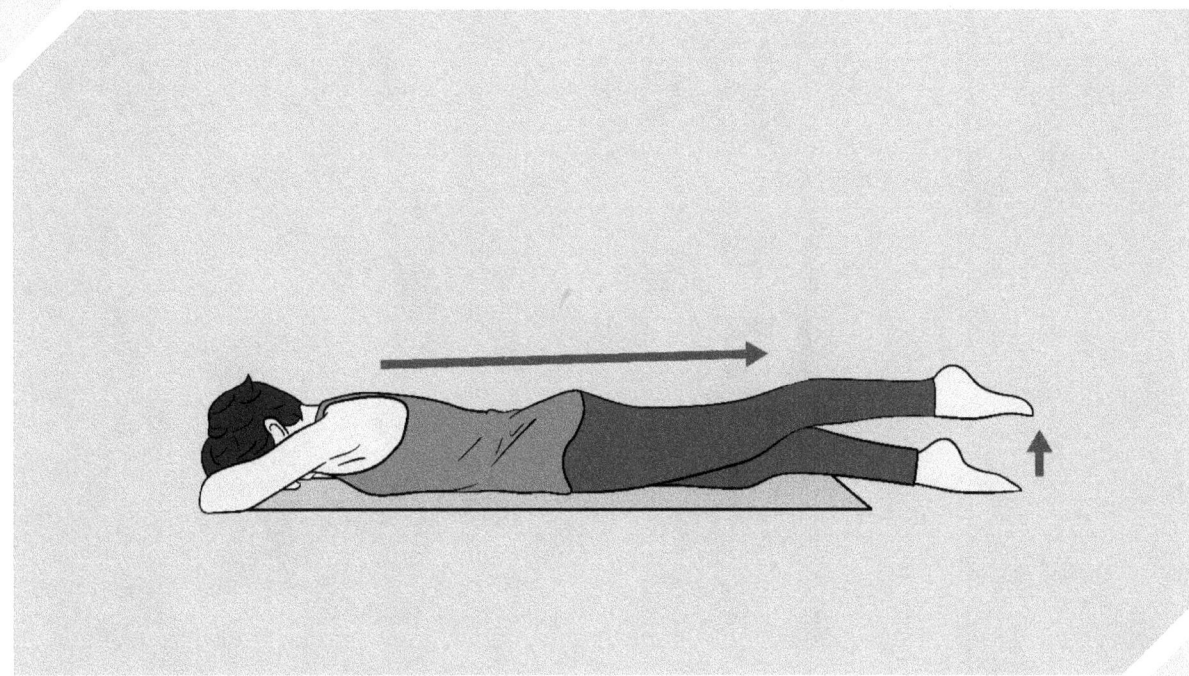

# PRONE LEG LIFTS

**Time Needed:** Two minutes

## Directions:

1. Lay face down on a padded mat. Legs should be straight and hands down by your thighs.

2. Engage your core and glutes as you lift your right leg off the mat a few inches. Try to get your thigh lifted off the floor but keep your pelvis glued to the mat. Lower your leg to the starting position. Repeat this leg a total of 10 times.

3. Switch legs and lift your left leg off the mat for 10 repetitions.

**Cautions:** Keep your neck from straining by keeping it long and lengthened as you gaze down towards the mat.

**Level Up:** Increase the number of reps.

**Benefits:** Targets the glutes and lower back for strengthening.

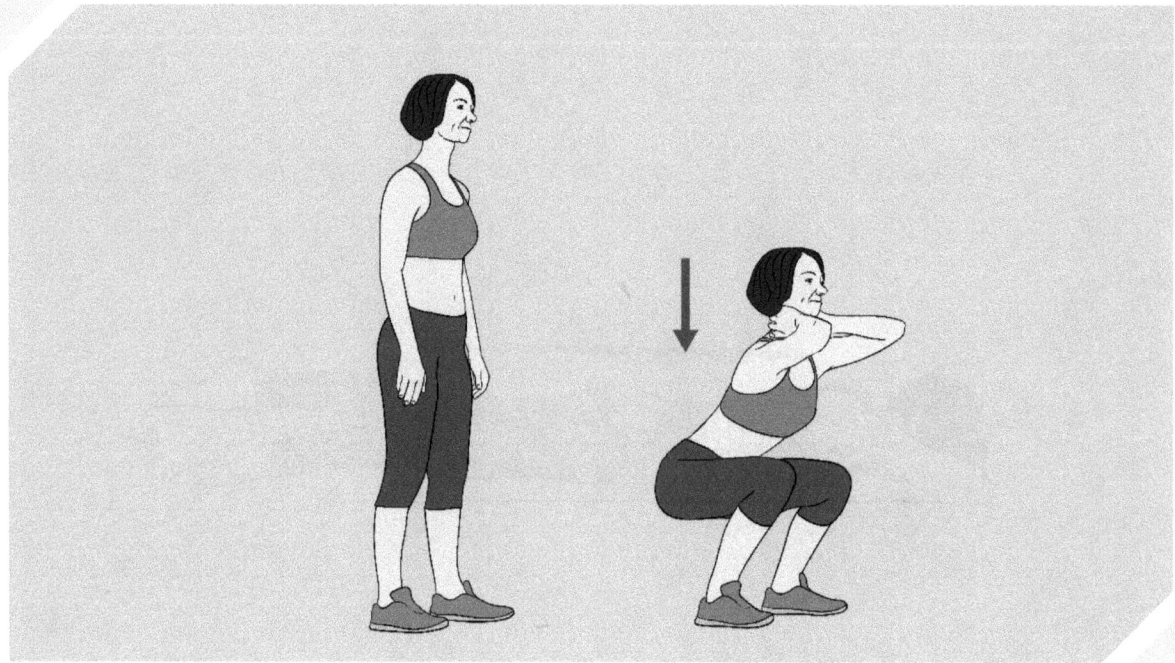

# SQUATS

## Time Needed: One minute

## Directions:

1.  Stand up tall next to a countertop or sturdy chair. Place one or both hands on the chair for support. Feet should be a hip-width distance apart.

2.  Keep your upper body upright as you bend at the knees and keep your feet flat on the floor. Move your buttocks back as if you were going to sit down and lower as far as you can comfortably. Squeeze your glutes as you rise back up to starting position.

3.  Repeat for 20 reps.

**Cautions:** Watch your balance as you do the squats. Only go down as far as you are able. As you get stronger you can increase how deep you squat.

**Level Up:** Place your hands on your hips or behind your head to make this more challenging. You can also add weights to both hands.

**Benefits:** Works and strengthens the major muscles of your lower body: glutes, quads, and hamstrings.

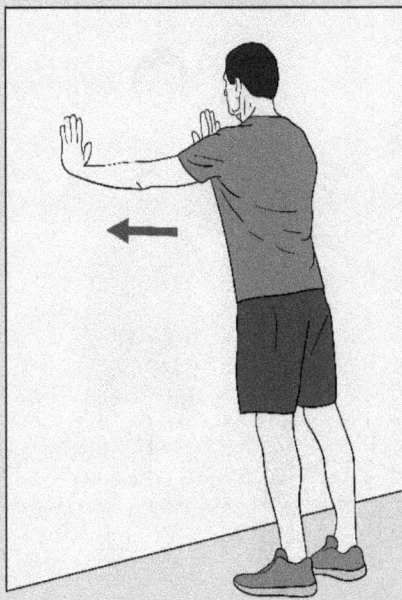

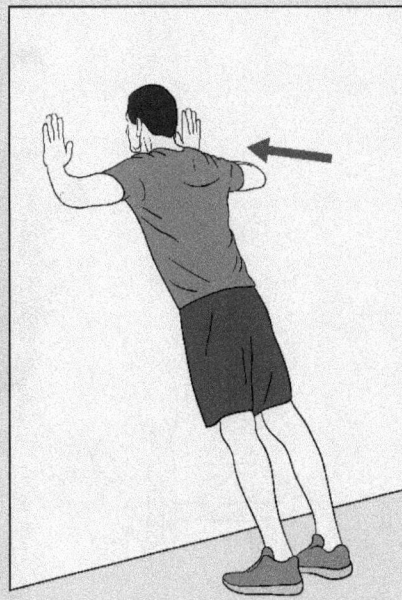

# Standing Push-Up

## Time Needed: Two minutes

## Directions:

1. Stand up straight with your arms straight out in front of you and palms flat against a wall. Hands should be the same height as your shoulders.

2. Don't move your feet. Bend both elbows and move your face and chest towards the wall. Keep your back and legs straight. Your shoulders, hips, knees, and ankles should form a diagonal line. Slowly push back to the starting position.

3. Repeat the standing push-up a total of 20 times, taking a break if you need to.

**Cautions:** Don't hurry through the exercise or use momentum. Slow and controlled movements are best.

**Level Up:** To make this harder, step a little further away from the wall.

**Benefits:** Strengthens your chest, core, upper back, and arm muscles.

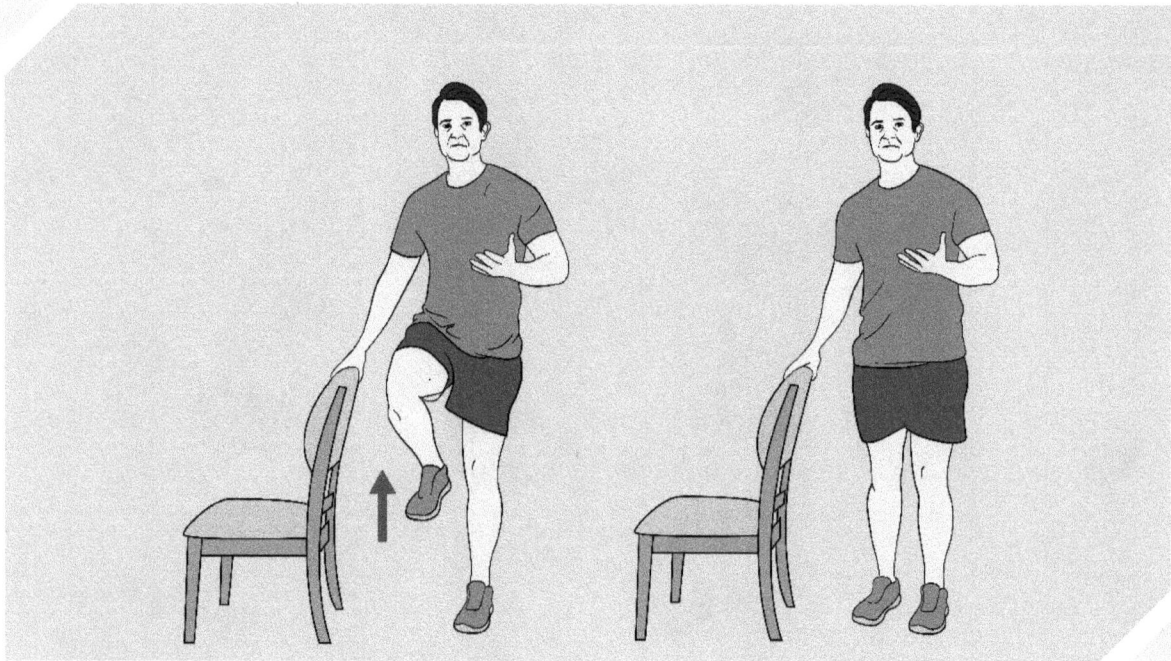

# STOMPING

**Time Needed:** One minute

## Directions:

1. Stand up tall next to a countertop or sturdy chair with one hand on it for support. Feet should be a hip-width distance apart.

2. Lift your right knee to hip height and stomp your right foot down on the ground as if you were crushing a bug or can beneath it. Repeat for a total of 10 times.

3. Switch legs. Lift your left knee to hip height and now stomp your left foot down on the ground 10 times.

**Cautions:** Be careful to stomp with a flexed foot so that your entire foot comes down on the floor at the same time (not toes or heel first).

**Level Up:** Increase the number of reps.

**Benefits:** This is an impact-loading exercise that can help build bone density in your ankles and hips.

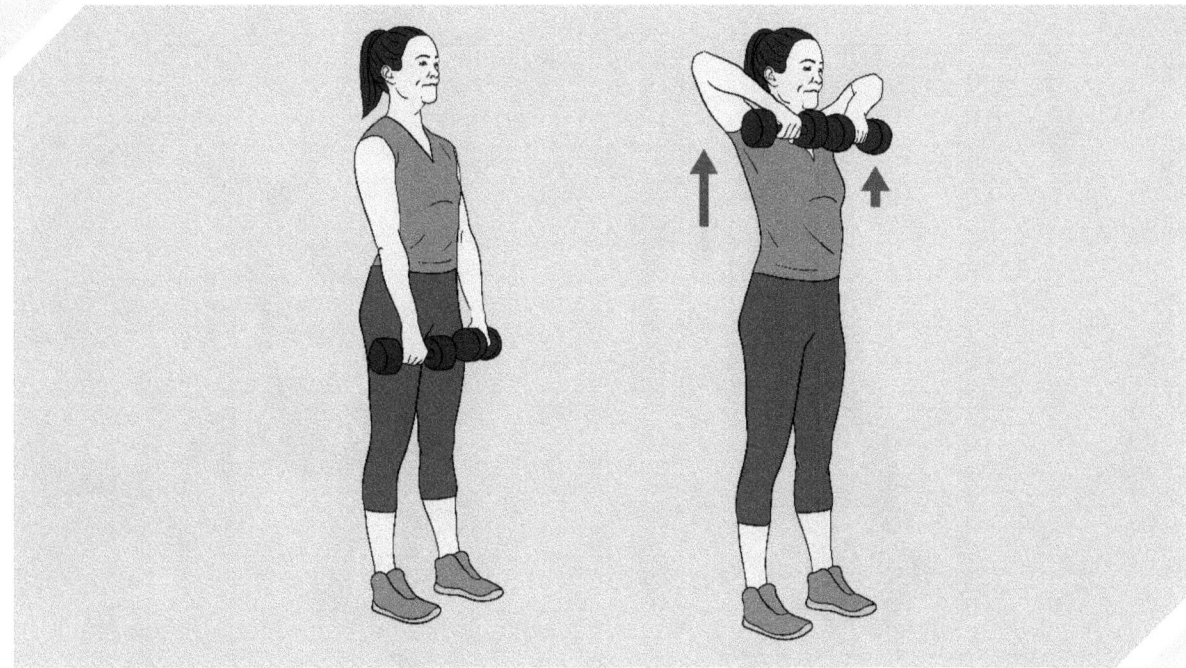

# UPRIGHT ROWS

**Time Needed:** Two minutes

## Directions:

1. Stand up tall with your feet a hip-width distance apart. Hold water bottles or light hand weights in your hands.

2. Straighten your arms and place your hands in front of you with weights resting on the front of your hips. Bend your elbows out to the sides as you raise the weights up towards your chin. Slowly lower weights back down to the starting position.

3. Repeat for 10 reps.

**Cautions:** Do not lift your shoulders as you lift the weights up towards your chin. Keep your shoulders pressed down and away from your ears.

**Level Up:** To make this more challenging, increase the number of reps or increase the amount of weight you are using.

**Benefits:** Helps to increase upper back and upper arm strength.

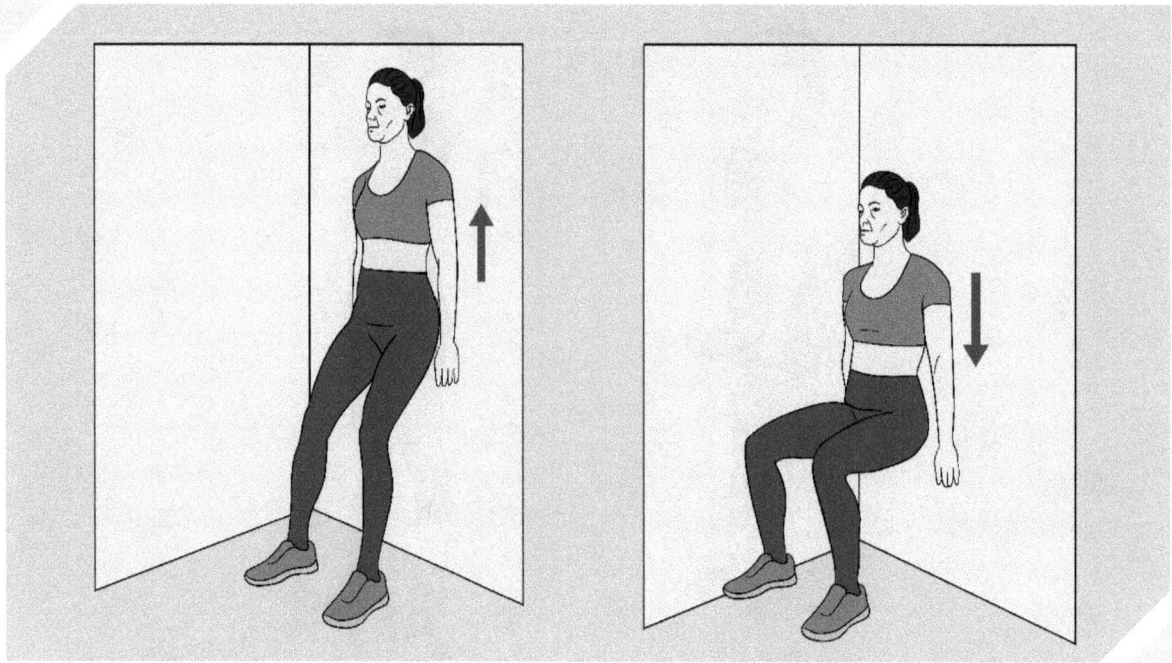

# WALL SLIDE

## Time Needed: One minute

## Directions:

1. Stand up tall with your shoulders, back, and buttocks against a wall. Your feet should be a hip-width distance apart and your heels a few inches away from the wall.

2. Place your palms on the wall and allow your body to slowly slide down the wall into a supported squat with your head, back, and buttocks in contact with the wall. Slowly slide back up to the starting position.

3. Repeat the wall slide a total of 10 times.

**Cautions:** When first starting out, only slide down a few inches or until you can comfortably slide back up.

**Level Up:** As your legs get stronger, you can go deeper into the slide and increase reps.

**Benefits:** Engages core and back muscles while strengthening quads.

# Chapter 5:
# Improving Your Cardio

This chapter is going to be a little different than the previous ones. We are going to outline some things you can do to improve your cardiovascular system. How does that relate to bone health?

Any type of movement that increases your heart rate is a benefit to heart health and circulatory health. Aerobic weight-bearing exercises also engage the bones,

> " *A cardio workout increases blood flow and acts as a filter system. It brings nutrients like oxygen, protein, and iron to the muscles that you've been training and helps them recover faster.*
>
> **Harley Pasternak** "

muscles, and tendons throughout your body while strengthening your heart and lungs.

If you have osteoporosis or osteopenia, you want to be careful of the exercises you choose to do. Depending on your situation, you will need to modify exercises or skip them altogether. As always, check with your doctor before adding an exercise to your routine.

In general, if you have osteoporosis, there are certain cardio exercises to avoid, including downhill skiing, golf, high-impact aerobics, jump rope, running, skating, and tennis. Any type of movement that involves jerking, twisting, sudden changes of direction or heightened potential for falls is not recommended for those with brittle or weakened bones.

The good news? There are still so many ways to fit cardio into your daily routine!

Listed below are 12 ways to develop your cardiovascular system and get your heart pumping. Each exercise is described, plus ideas on where and how long they can be performed. Some of them require equipment while others do not. They are all osteoporosis-friendly, with modifications. Some things included on this list may surprise you!

# CARDIO EXERCISES

The first six exercises are very common recommendations for weight-bearing exercises by the ortho and osteoporosis community as being safe for those with weakened bones. There are, however, still precautions you must take when participating in these. Remember to warm up for 5 to 10 minutes before doing any cardio exercises.

Following the list of common exercises are some not-so-common ones that are also great weight-bearing exercises. Some of these require equipment or access to a gym.

# Common Weight-bearing Exercises

## Dancing

**Examples:** Ballroom, line dancing, swing, and zumba classes at the gym or community center. Also can be done at home, with or without a partner.

**Time Needed:** 10 to 30 minutes, three times a week.

**Cautions:** Be aware of any turns or movements that may cause you to bump into others or potentially fall.

**Benefits:** Increases heart rate and engages muscles through music and movement. Provides odd-impact loading exercise for the bones. Can be done alone at home or in a fun social situation.

## Elliptical

**Examples:** Elliptical machines at the gym or at home can be adjusted for resistance and speed.

**Time Needed:** 10 to 30 minutes, three times a week.

**Cautions:** Hold onto handlebars for support and to work out the upper body. Be aware of pinch hazards where the handles attach to the machine.

**Benefits:** Raises heart rate for a total body workout that is easy on the joints.

## Hiking

**Examples:** Hike in nearby parks, trails, or hills.

**Time Needed:** 20 to 40 minutes, three times a week.

**Cautions:** Wear the right kind of shoes and stick to groomed trails to avoid getting lost or potential trip hazards. It is wise to use the buddy system and hike with a friend or group. Use a hiking stick or poles for added stability.

**Benefits:** Gets your heart rate up while letting you enjoy the fresh air, outdoors, and sunshine. Plus, it's free.

## Low-impact Aerobics

**Examples:** At-home videos, online classes, or gym classes are all available.

**Time Needed:** 20 to 40 minutes, three times a week.

**Cautions:** Be mindful to practice good form. These exercises usually are done to music which can get you going but don't turn it into high-impact.

**Benefits:** Strengthens you cardiovascularly while being easy on the joints. Is also an odd-impact loading exercise. Can be done alone at home or at the gym for social interaction.

## Stair Stepper or Stair Climbing

**Examples:** Stair-step machines at the gym or a flight of stairs in your home, apartment building, or the local mall.

**Time Needed:** 10 to 30 minutes, three times a week.

**Cautions:** Be sure to watch your posture and not lean too far forward when climbing stairs. Lift your foot high enough to avoid tripping and place your whole foot on the step. Hold on to the rails for support.

**Benefits:** Increases heart rate while targeting the lower body and strengthening legs.

## Walking

**Examples:** Treadmills at the gym or home. Walking outside in your neighborhood or park. You can change the pace or change directions (walk laterally or backward using caution) to increase intensity. Walking poles, like Nordic poles, can be used to also work the upper body.

**Time Needed:** 20 to 40 minutes, three times a week.

**Cautions:** Be aware of tripping hazards. Use walking poles for support.

**Benefits:** Gentle way to increase heart rate. It can be done for free anytime and almost anywhere.

# Less Common Weight-bearing Exercises

The next five weight-bearing exercises are not as commonly recommended but can be osteoporosis-friendly when done correctly.

## Boxing

**Examples:** Boxing classes and heavy punching bags at the gym. Personal heavy bags can be purchased for home use.

**Time Needed:** 10 to 30 minutes, three times a week.

**Cautions:** Be sure to wear hand wraps and boxing gloves to protect hands and wrists. It is recommended you receive instruction from a trainer before beginning a boxing routine to learn proper form and avoid injury.

**Benefits:** A good cardio workout that engages the whole body, mainly the upper body and core. Because this exercise is impact loading for the upper body, boxing increases bone density in the wrist and shoulder joints.

## CrossFit Training

**Examples:** CrossFit classes at the gym involve a combination of aerobic exercise, weight training, and plyometrics.

**Time Needed:** 20 to 40 minutes, three times a week.

**Cautions:** It is important to consult your doctor and a CrossFit Trainer on specific exercise modifications and proper techniques when doing a CrossFit program to avoid injury. While some people may think this program is too aggressive, there are elements of it that are osteoporosis-friendly with modifications.

**Benefits:** Increases muscle strength through odd-impact loading exercises while providing an aerobic workout.

## Cross-country Skiing

**Examples:** Cross-country skiing is done outdoors in the snow or on indoor machines like NordicTrack at the gym or at home.

**Time Needed:** 20 to 40 minutes, three times a week.

**Cautions:** If you are a first-time skier, get instructions on the proper technique used in this type of skiing. When skiing outdoors stick to groomed trails, watch for inclement weather, and use the buddy system to avoid getting lost or stranded.

**Benefits:** Increases heart rate while providing a full-body workout. If done outdoors, enjoy the fresh air and scenery.

## Rowing

**Examples:** Rowing machines at the gym or at home.

**Time Needed:** 10 to 30 minutes, three times a week.

**Cautions:** It is important to use good technique and be cautious of leaning too far forward or rounding your back. This is a safe exercise if done correctly, so it is recommended to have a trainer instruct you in the proper form.

**Benefits:** Raises the heart rate and works 86% of the muscles in the body. This exercise also strengthens the spine and the muscles surrounding it.

### *Stationary Bike (standing)*

**Examples:** Upright stationary bike at the gym or home ridden while standing up. Take note that this does not include recumbent bikes since sitting is not weight-bearing.

**Time Needed:** 20 to 40 minutes, three times a week.

**Cautions:** If your stationary bike has shoe cages, be sure that they are snug around your foot or that your spin shoes are snapped in correctly before standing. There needs to be enough tension on the bike that it is an effort to push down on the pedals otherwise it is not weight-bearing.

**Benefits:** Quickly gets your heart rate up and targets lower body strengthening while being easy on the joints.

# One More Thing

One last exercise to consider is vibration plate therapy. Technically it is not a cardio exercise, but it is worth mentioning. There is ongoing research on the benefits of vibration plate therapy. Currently, there is not any conclusive evidence yet that shows it helps build bone density. However, it has been shown in some trials to improve overall balance and shows the potential to be helpful for those with osteoporosis.

### *Vibration Plate Therapy*

**Examples:** Vibration plates are available at the gym or can be purchased for at-home use.

**Time Needed:** 15 to 30 minutes, three times a week.

**Cautions:** Hold on to handrails for support. If you feel dizzy at any time, shut off the machine.

**Benefits:** Forces your muscles to contract and relax many times through vibrations transmitted throughout your body and can help improve overall balance.

# Part 3:
## The Action Plan

> *When you look at people who are successful, you will find that they aren't the people who are motivated but have consistency in their motivation.*
>
> **Arsene Wenger**

# Chapter 6:
# Exercise Routines

We have covered a lot of exercise options in many different areas including balance, flexibility, posture, strength, and cardio. Wondering where to start and what to do? Don't worry—we've got you covered!

Getting started on any exercise routine requires a decision and ongoing determination. You are already on the path because you are reading this book. Now it is time to put your knowledge into action.

> *With consistency and reps and routine you're going to achieve your goals and get where you want to be.*
>
> **Mandy Rose**

Before you do any exercises, remember to consult with your doctor or a medical professional that is familiar with your health history and any pre-existing conditions you may have. Taking this book to your doctor's appointment can give them an idea of the exercises you are planning to do and at what intensity level. They may suggest making certain modifications specific to you and your circumstances.

This chapter is devoted to getting you started on your 30-day journey to better bone health. Four weeks of consistent activity can help build a habit that lasts a lifetime.

How the month is broken down:

✧ Each week features a 3-2 combo of targeted exercises and cardio. Some weeks you will have two days of cardio and the following week you will have three days of cardio. Same with training exercises.

✧ The exercises are arranged into five days of movement and two days of rest.

This allows you to pick your rest days since everyone's schedule is different. You may decide to take the weekend off because you are visiting with family or you might choose to take one day off in the middle of the week and one day off on the weekend.

◇ Each day will include a combination of exercises in balance, flexibility, posture, strength, or cardio. There is lots of variety to ensure you don't get bored.

Remember to take five to ten minutes to warm up your body before starting any exercise, whether it is training or cardio. Warming up increases the flow of blood to your muscles and increases your body temperature (that's why it's called warming up!). Muscles are less prone to injury and less likely to get as sore when warmed up. And after you are done? Take five to ten minutes to cool down. Exercise can raise your heart rate and your blood pressure, so you want to take the time to bring those back down to a normal rate before going on with the rest of your day.

There are some good ideas for warming up and cooling down.

◇ **Warm Up**: Walking in place, raising arms overhead, low-impact jumping jacks, or any movement that increases your breath rate and gets your blood moving.

◇ **Cool Down**: Walking in place until heart rate goes down, slow overhead stretch, or any slow and controlled motions that allow your breathing and heart rate to return to normal.

Let's get started!

# Week 1: Three Days Training and Two Days CardioYou choose your two rest days.

## *Day 1*

**Warm Up and Cool Down:** 5 to 10 minutes for each

**Balance:** 3 Way Hip Kick, Bird Dog

**Flexibility:** Breaststroke, Calf Stretch, Chest Stretch

**Posture:** Dead Bug, Glute Bridge

**Strength:** Clamshell, Elbow Side Extensions, Forearm Plank

## *Day 2*

**Warm Up and Cool Down:** 5 to 10 minutes for each

**Cardio:** Twenty minutes of cardio. Ideas include dancing, elliptical, or hiking.

## *Day 3*

**Warm Up and Cool Down:** 5 to 10 minutes for each

**Balance:** Foot Taps, Head Rotation, Heel Raises

**Flexibility:** Corner Stretch, Inner Thigh Stretch, Kneeling Hip Flexor Stretch

**Posture:** Head Press, Isometric Abdominals

**Strength:** Hammer Curls, Hamstring Curls

## *Day 4*

**Warm Up and Cool Down:** 5 to 10 minutes for each

**Cardio:** 30 minutes of a different cardio than the one you did earlier this week. Ideas include low-impact aerobics, stair stepping, or walking.

## *Day 5*

**Warm Up and Cool Down:** 5 to 10 minutes for each

**Balance:** Hip Abductor, Lateral Stepping

**Flexibility:** One Leg Kick, Prone Heel Squeeze

**Posture:** Modified Forearm Side Plank, Shoulder Blade Squeeze, Shoulder Rolls

**Strength:** Lateral Shoulder Raise, Prone Leg Lifts

# Week 2: Three Days Cardio and Two Days Training

Remember, you choose your two rest days.

## *Day 1*

**Warm Up and Cool Down:** 5 to 10 minutes for each**Cardio:** 20 minutes of cardio. Ideas include boxing, CrossFit training, cross-country skiing, or rowing.

## *Day 2*

**Warm Up and Cool Down:** 5 to 10 minutes for each

**Balance:** Mini Lunge, Over the Shoulder Walk, Single Leg Stance

**Flexibility:** Side Angle Pose, Side Kick

**Posture:** Tandem Stand, Tandem Walk

**Strength:** Squats, Standing Push-up

## *Day 3*

**Warm Up and Cool Down:** 5 to 10 minutes for each

**Cardio:** 30 minutes of cardio, different from what you did earlier this week. Ideas include stationary bike riding while standing, dancing, or elliptical.

## *Day 4*

**Warm Up and Cool Down:** 5 to 10 minutes for each

**Balance:** Sit to Stand, Standing Marches

**Flexibility:** Superman Pose, Supine Hand-to-Big Toe

**Posture:** Tree Pose, Wall Angel, Waxing

**Strength:** Stomping, Upright Rows, Wall Slide

## *Day 5*

**Warm Up and Cool Down:** 5 to 10 minutes for each

**Cardio:** 20 minutes of cardio, different from what you did already this week. Ideas include elliptical or walking.

# Week 3: Three Days Training and Two Days Cardio

Remember, you choose your two rest days.

## *Day 1*

**Warm Up and Cool Down:** 5 to 10 minutes for each

**Balance:** 3 Way Hip Kick, Bird Dog

**Flexibility:** Breaststroke, Calf Stretch, Chest Stretch

**Posture:** Dead Bug, Glute Bridge

**Strength:** Clamshell, Elbow Side Extension, Forearm Plank

## *Day 2*

**Warm Up and Cool Down:** 5 to 10 minutes for each**Cardio:** 30 minutes of cardio. Ideas include CrossFit training, low-impact aerobics or stair stepping.

## *Day 3*

**Warm Up and Cool Down:** 5 to 10 minutes for each

**Balance:** Foot Taps, Head Rotation, Heel Raises

**Flexibility:** Corner Stretch, Inner Thigh Stretch, Kneeling Hip Flexor Stretch

**Posture:** Head Press, Isometric Abdominals

**Strength:** Hammer Curls, Hamstring Curls

## *Day 4*

**Warm Up and Cool Down:** 5 to 10 minutes for each

**Cardio:** 40 minutes of cardio, different from what you did earlier this week. Ideas include dancing, hiking, or cross-country skiing.

## Day 5

**Warm Up and Cool Down:** 5 to 10 minutes for each

**Balance:** Hip Abductor, Lateral Stepping

**Flexibility:** One Leg Kick, Prone Heel Squeeze

**Posture:** Modified Forearm Side Plank, Shoulder Blade Squeeze, Shoulder Rolls

**Strength:** Lateral Shoulder Raise, Prone Leg Lifts

# Week 4: Three Days Cardio and Two Days Training

Remember, you choose your two rest days.

## Day 1

**Warm Up and Cool Down:** 5 to 10 minutes for each

**Cardio:** 30 minutes of cardio. Ideas include boxing, rowing, or stationary bike riding while standing.

## Day 2

**Warm Up and Cool Down:** 5 to 10 minutes for each

**Balance:** Mini Lunge, Over the Shoulder Walk, Single Leg Stance

**Flexibility:** Side Angle Pose, Side Kick

**Posture:** Tandem Stand, Tandem Walk

**Strength:** Squats, Standing Push-up

## Day 3

**Warm Up and Cool Down:** 5 to 10 minutes for each**Cardio:** 40 minutes of cardio, different from what you did earlier this week. Ideas include dancing and walking.

## Day 4

**Warm Up and Cool Down:** 5 to 10 minutes for each

**Balance:** Sit to Stand, Standing Marches

**Flexibility:** Superman Pose, Supine Hand-to-Big Toe

**Posture:** Tree Pose, Wall Angel, Waxing

**Strength:** Stomping, Upright Rows, Wall Slide

## Day 5

**Warm Up and Cool Down:** 5 to 10 minutes for each

**Cardio:** 30 minutes of cardio, different from what you've already done this week. Ideas include elliptical, low-impact aerobics, or hiking.

# Conclusion

You made it! Here we are at the end of the book. Are you proud of yourself for reading it? I'm proud of you. By recognizing your motivation and goal to achieve better health, you have learned so much along the way.

Think about it. You have become more educated on bone disease, bone health (you will always remember osteoblasts!), the risk factors, and the effects of osteoporosis. What's even more important is you also know how critical good nutrition and good exercise are to preventing and reducing bone loss. With this added knowledge, now you can better advocate for yourself, a family member, a friend, a patient, or someone you care for when interacting with general practitioners, endocrinologists, orthopedic specialists, and other healthcare professionals that are providing care. Having seen the consequences of osteoporosis in the life of someone I care for, I know from personal experience how devastating a bone disease can be when knowledge is lacking.

The importance of exercise, especially resistance training and weight-bearing exercises, can't be stressed enough. There's no getting away from it. Exercise is necessary for better bones. Aren't you glad you learned that different physical skills like balance, flexibility, posture, strength, and cardio can be improved by exercise?

In Chapter 1, we covered how to improve your balance. A loss of balance can cause us to fall, trip, and possibly fracture bones. Because balance and stability are necessary for every day movements like going up and down staircases, getting in and out of cars, and even reaching for that glass on your kitchen shelf, we want to be sure that we maintain and strengthen the muscles that support our ability to stay upright.

Chapter 2 was all about flexibility. When our muscles are tight and stiff, our flexibility and stretchiness decreases. This causes pain and possible imbalance in our bodies. The exercises in this chapter addressed our need to keep our muscles, tendons, and joints limber through gentle stretches that can be done on a regular basis.

Improving your posture was the focus of Chapter 3. It isn't just for beauty queens! Good posture is for everyone who wants to protect their back and spine from pain, prevent breathing difficulties, and pursue a more confident attitude. Standing up straight requires strong core muscles throughout the torso and the exercises featured were designed to help strengthen those muscles.

In Chapter 4, we talked about building your strength. Muscles lose mass and decrease in strength with age. But we need them more than ever as we age. Strong muscles are important in order for us to complete the daily tasks to care for ourselves and continue to live and thrive in our independence. The exercises in this section concentrated on building strength in the large muscles of the body like the legs and arms, as well as improving grip and wrist strength.

Chapter 5 highlighted all the fun things to keep moving and work our cardiovascular system. Were you surprised by some of the exercises? The common weight-bearing exercises are ones that can be done almost anywhere with some requiring equipment readily accessible at any gym. The not-so-common exercises offered some interesting and exciting possibilities for other ways to get in some heart healthy movement. A strong cardiovascular system is important for our bodies in order to ward off illness, maintain a healthy weight, and to recharge our minds.

We put it all together in Chapter 6 with an action plan. The exercise routines provided offer a blueprint to follow for each day and each week of the month. We've all heard the saying that Rome was not built in a day. Well, neither are our bodies. It takes consistency, persistence, and maybe a little bit of crazy to keep going. Results take time, but with a month's worth of varied exercises laid out in a plan, those results are more likely to appear. Friends, this is not the end of your journey. It is just the beginning. You are equipped now to prevent further bone loss, build back healthy bone tissue, and stay on the path to more fulfilling physical health. Our hope and prayer is that you enjoy the journey and enjoy the results you will earn through your diligence. I encourage you not to wait any longer. Better bone health is just ahead!

If this book has provided you with a good overview of osteoporosis and its effects, a solution to building better bones through resistance training and weight-bearing exercise, and an action plan that you can start upon, please consider leaving us a review. I would love to know how it has helped you or your loved one, and I thank you in advance.

# Scan the QR Code below to leave a review:

*I hope you enjoy good health and happiness on the long road ahead of you, and I wish you all the best. Thank you for allowing me to share my knowledge with you.*

Baz Thompson

# References

ABC Pilates. (2015, September 14). *Try this: Pilates breaststroke*. Abcfitstudio.com. https://abcfitstudio.com/trythis-breaststroke/

ACE Fitness. (n.d.). *Exercise Library: kneeling hip-flexor stretch*. Www.acefitness.org. https://www.acefitness.org/resources/everyone/exercise-library/142/kneeling-hip-flexor-stretch/

AlgaeCal, G. (2018, November 2). *5 best shoulder exercises for osteoporosis*. AlgaeCal. https://blog.algaecal.com/best-shoulder-exercises/

Arthritis New South Wales. (2019, November 18). *Shoulder blade squeeze | Arthritis NSW*. Www.arthritisnsw.org.au. https://www.arthritisnsw.org.au/exercise-shoulder-blade-squeeze/

Bedosky, L. (2021, March 13). *The best core exercises for seniors*. Get Healthy U | Chris Freytag. https://gethealthyu.com/best-core-exercises-for-seniors/

Bodysmart Health. (2020, January 9). *Osteoporosis: What exercise is best?* BodySmart Health +. https://bodysmarthealth.com.au/osteoporosis-what-exercise-is-best/

Bone Health and Osteoporosis Foundation. (n.d.). *Exercise to stay healthy*. Bone Health & Osteoporosis Foundation. https://www.bonehealthandosteoporosis.org/preventing-fractures/exercise-to-stay-healthy/

Brainy Quote. (n.d.-a). *Arsene Wenger quotes*. BrainyQuote. Retrieved October 26, 2022, from https://www.brainyquote.com/quotes/arsene_wenger_598799?src=t_consistency

Brainy Quote. (n.d.-b). *Dr. Seuss quotes*. BrainyQuote. Retrieved October 26, 2022, from https://www.brainyquote.com/quotes/dr_seuss_597903

Brainy Quote. (n.d.-c). *Harley Pasternak quotes*. BrainyQuote. Retrieved October 26, 2022, from https://www.brainyquote.com/quotes/harley_pasternak_938190?src=t_cardio

Brainy Quote. (n.d.-d). *Lee Haney quotes*. BrainyQuote. Retrieved October 26, 2022, from https://www.brainyquote.com/quotes/lee_haney_295632?src=t_exercise

Brainy Quote. (n.d.-e). *Mandy Rose quotes*. BrainyQuote. Retrieved October 26, 2022, from https://www.brainyquote.com/quotes/mandy_rose_1104677?src=t_consistency

Brainy Quote. (n.d.-f). *Richard Simmons quotes*. BrainyQuote. Retrieved October 26, 2022, from https://www.brainyquote.com/quotes/richard_simmons_417270

Brainy Quote. (n.d.-g). *Samantha Stosur quotes.* BrainyQuote. Retrieved October 26, 2022, from https://www.brainyquote.com/quotes/samantha_stosur_475948

Brainy Quote. (2019). *Benjamin Franklin quotes.* BrainyQuote; BrainyQuote. https://www.brainyquote.com/quotes/benjamin_franklin_141119

Brown, R. (2022, January 19). *How to keep skiing pain-free into middle age and beyond.* Next Avenue. https://www.nextavenue.org/how-to-keep-skiing-pain-free/

Davidson, K. (2021, December 6). *Wall pushups: How to do this modified pushup variation.* Healthline. https://www.healthline.com/health/fitness-exercise/wall-pushups

Dumain, T. (2019, August 30). *Osteoporosis exercise: moves to strengthen bones and prevent fractures.* CreakyJoints. https://creakyjoints.org/diet-exercise/osteoporosis-exercises/

Fetters, K. A. (2018, November 27). *6 best balance exercises for better stability.* SilverSneakers. https://www.silversneakers.com/blog/balance-exercises-seniors/Fetters, K. A. (2019, March 12). *6 core exercises to ease lower back pain.* SilverSneakers. https://www.silversneakers.com/blog/core-exercises-ease-back-pain/

Fraticelli, T. (2019, May 19). *12 balance exercises for seniors | with printable pictures and PDF.* PTProgress | Career Development, Education, Health. https://www.ptprogress.com/balance-exercises-for-seniors/

Frey, M. (2022, July 28). *How to do hammer curls: proper form, variations, and common mistakes.* Verywell Fit. https://www.verywellfit.com/how-to-hammer-curls-techniques-benefits-variations-4788329

Freytag, C. (n.d.). *How to do modified forearm side plank.* Get Healthy U | Chris Freytag. Retrieved October 24, 2022, from https://gethealthyu.com/exercise/modified-forearm-side-plank/

Gerace, J. (2007). *Exercise for osteoporosis.* WebMD; WebMD. https://www.webmd.com/osteoporosis/features/exercise-for-osteoporosis

Gigney, G. (2021, July 9). *30 weight training quotes that are sure to motivate you.* Www.gym-Pact.com. https://www.gym-pact.com/weight-training-quotes

Gulbrandson, D. (2019, January 31). *Which weight bearing activities build bone in adults?* Herman & Wallace Pelvic Rehabilitation Continuing Education. https://hermanwallace.com/blog/which-weight-bearing-activities-build-bone-in-adults

Hall, D. (2017). *Shall we dance? Why we should all be dancing for our bones.* Theros.org.uk; Royal Osteoporosis Society. https://theros.org.uk/latest-news/2017-12-21-shall-we-dance-why-we-should-all-be-dancing-for-our-bones/

Higgs, J., Derbyshire, E., & Styles, K. (2017). Nutrition and osteoporosis prevention for the orthopaedic surgeon. *EFORT Open Reviews, 2*(6), 300–308. https://doi.org/10.1302/2058-5241.2.160079

Ippoliti, A. (2017, September 28). *Master reclining hand-to-big toe pose in 5 steps.* Yoga Journal. https://www.yogajournal.com/poses/master-reclining-hand-to-big-toe-pose/

Jones, H. (2021, November 4). *What are the benefits of yoga for osteoporosis?* Verywell Health. https://www.verywellhealth.com/the-health-benefits-of-yoga-for-osteoporosis-5203363

Kenway, M. (2022, March 11). *2 osteoporosis exercises for hips at home (video)| prolapse safe - pelvic exercises.* Pelvic Exercises Physiotherapy. https://www.pelvicexercises.com.au/osteoporosis-exercises-for-hips-at-home/?v=7516fd43adaa&c=cf13ce20305c

Kutcher, M. (n.d.). *The best exercises for stronger bones (osteoporosis exercises).* More Life Health - Seniors Health & Fitness. Retrieved October 25, 2022, from https://morelifehealth.com/articles/strong-bones-part3

Laliberte, M. (2019, January 30). *This is how long your skeleton takes to regenerate itself.* The Healthy. https://www.thehealthy.com/osteoporosis/bones-constantly-regenerate/

Laskowski, E. (n.d.). *Is whole-body vibration an effective workout?* Mayo Clinic. https://www.mayoclinic.org/healthy-lifestyle/fitness/expert-answers/whole-body-vibration/faq-20057958#:~:text=Advocates%20say%20that%20as%20little

Leonard, J. (2021, March 25). *10 benefits of cross country skiing for seniors (2022)*. Impowerage.com. https://impowerage.com/benefits-of-cross-country-skiing/

Limited, G. P. (2022, May 8). *Hammer curls vs normal curls*. Gym Plan. https://gymplanapp.com/hammer-curls-vs-normal-curls/

Lohr, R. (2015, April 15). *Try Nordic walking*. SeniorsSkiing.com. https://www.seniorsskiing.com/try-nordic-walking-many-benefits-by-adding-poles-to-hike/

Mayo Clinic. (n.d.). *Strength training: Get stronger, leaner, healthier*. Mayo Clinic. https://www.mayoclinic.org/healthy-lifestyle/fitness/in-depth/strength-training/art-20046670#:~:text=Strength%20training%20may%20enhance%20yourMedical Guardian. (2013, October 28). *The best (and worst) exercises for osteoporosis*. Medical Guardian. https://www.medicalguardian.com/medical-alert-blog/fitness/the-best-and-worst-exercises-for-osteoporosis

Nall, R. (2017, January 25). *Living with osteoporosis: 8 exercises to strengthen your bones*. Healthline. https://www.healthline.com/health/managing-osteoporosis/exercises-to-strengthen-your-bones#Exercises-to-avoid

National Library of Medicine. (2019). *The burden of bone disease*. Nih.gov; Office of the Surgeon General (US). https://www.ncbi.nlm.nih.gov/books/NBK45502/

*Osteoporosis exercise: Weight-Bearing and muscle strengthening exercises osteoporosis exercise: Balance, posture and functional exercises*. (2017). https://www.sanfordhealth.org/-/media/org/files/patient-education/019053-00137-booklet-exercise-balancepdf?la=en&hash=B1ACF51C0B3BD2733DB09C0C6F80A51CE49327CA

Pilates Anytime. (n.d.). *One leg kick with Kristi Cooper - exercise 1435*. Pilates Anytime. Retrieved October 24, 2022, from https://www.pilatesanytime.com/exercise-view/1435/video/Pilates-One-Leg-Kick-by-Kristi-Cooper

Pilates Anytime. (2014). *Side kick with Adrianne Crawford - exercise 1438*. Pilates Anytime. https://www.pilatesanytime.com/exercise-view/1438/video/Pilates-Side-Kick-by-Adrianne-Crawford

Porter, J. L., & Varacallo, M. (2019, June 4). *Osteoporosis*. Nih.gov; StatPearls Publishing. https://www.ncbi.nlm.nih.gov/books/NBK441901/

Rally Fitness. (2016, October 26). *How CrossFit training can prevent and cure osteoporosis*. Rally Fitness LLC. https://rallyfitness.com/blogs/news/how-crossfit-training-can-prevent-and-cure-osteoporosis

Rathod, R. (2021, October 28). *12 safe exercises for osteoporosis with steps & pictures*. Stylecraze. https://www.stylecraze.com/articles/exercises-for-osteoporosis/

Schrift, D. (n.d.-a). *Calf muscle stretches for seniors and the elderly – ELDERGYM®*. Eldergym. https://eldergym.com/calf-muscle-stretches/

Schrift, D. (n.d.-b). *Shoulder muscle workout for seniors and the elderly – ELDERGYM®*. Eldergym. https://eldergym.com/shoulder-muscle-workout/

Schrift, D. (n.d.-c). *Stretching legs exercises for seniors and the elderly – ELDERGYM®*. Eldergym. https://eldergym.com/stretching-legs/

Schrift, D. (n.d.-d). *Upper arm exercises for seniors and the elderly – ELDERGYM®*. Eldergym. https://eldergym.com/upper-arm-exercises/

Sherrington, C., Dean, C., Blackman, K., Canning, C., & Allen, N. (2008). *Weight-bearing exercise for better balance (WEBB)*. http://www.webb.org.au/attachments/File/WEBB_draft_19.pdf

Stein, J. (2006, December 4). *Keep exercising those bones*. Los Angeles Times. https://www.latimes.com/health/la-he-ask4dec04-story.html

Stockett, S. (2017, July 12). *Prone heel squeeze to tone your tush!* Custom Pilates and Yoga. https://www.custompilatesandyoga.com/prone-heel-squeeze/

Straith, M. (2019, May 22). *Simple posture exercises for osteoporosis that make a difference*. AlgaeCal. https://blog.algaecal.com/posture-exercises-osteoporosis/

Sundh, D., Nilsson, M., Zoulakis, M., Pasco, C., Yilmaz, M., Kazakia, G. J., Hellgren, M., & Lorentzon, M.

(2018). High-Impact Mechanical Loading Increases Bone Material Strength in Postmenopausal Women-A 3-Month Intervention Study. *Journal of Bone and Mineral Research, 33*(7), 1242–1251. https://doi.org/10.1002/jbmr.3431

Tam, J. (n.d.). *Impact loading activities – Jason H. Tam, M.D.* Orthopaedic Sports Medicine. Retrieved October 27, 2022, from http://jhtammd.com/impact-loading-activities/Terpening, C., & Rieger, C. (2017). *Stand tall with osteoporosis thru pilates content of program.* https://www.upstate.edu/hospital/pdf/healthlink/pilate-and-osteoporosis-061917.pdf

UCLA Ergonomics. (2019, April 4). *Posture strengthening exercises.* Ergonomics. https://ergonomics.ucla.edu/injuries-and-prevention/stretches/exercises/posture-strengthening-exercises

Unique Health and Fitness. (2019, April 27). *Why flexibility is so significant as we age.* Www.uniquehealthandfitness.com. https://www.uniquehealthandfitness.com/why-flexibility-is-so-significant-as-we-age#:~:text=The%20Benefits%20Of%20Flexibility%20While

Weber-Rajek, M., Mieszkowski, J., Niespodziński, B., & Ciechanowska, K. (2015). Whole-body vibration exercise in postmenopausal osteoporosis. *Menopausal Review, 1,* 41–47. https://doi.org/10.5114/pm.2015.48679

WebMD. (2021, March 18). *What causes balance issues in older adults.* WebMD. https://www.webmd.com/healthy-aging/what-causes-balance-issues-in-older-adults

Weiss, C. (2022, May 19). *Mayo Clinic Q and A: Osteoporosis and a bone-healthy diet.* Mayo Clinic News Network. https://newsnetwork.mayoclinic.org/discussion/mayo-clinic-q-and-a-osteoporosis-and-a-bone-healthy-diet/

White, A. (2022, July 4). *How to do a sitting to standing exercise: 7 steps (with pictures).* WikiHow. https://www.wikihow.com/Do-a-Sitting-to-Standing-Exercise